Practical Patient Safety

By

John Reynard DM FRCS Urol

Consultant Urological Surgeon, Department of Urology
The Churchill Hospital, Oxford, UK
and
Honorary Consultant Urological Surgeon
The National Spinal Injuries Centre
Stoke Mandeville Hospital, Buckinghamshire UK

John Reynolds DPhil FRCP

Consultant Physician and Clinical Pharmacologist,
John Radcliffe Hospital, Oxford

Peter Stevenson

Commercial Airline Pilot and
Honorary Patient Safety Lecturer,
Nuffield Department of Surgery, University of Oxford

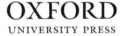

OXFORD
UNIVERSITY PRESS

OXFORD
UNIVERSITY PRESS

Great Clarendon Street, Oxford OX2 6DP

Oxford University Press is a department of the University of Oxford.
It furthers the University's objective of excellence in research, scholarship,
and education by publishing worldwide in

Oxford New York

Auckland Cape Town Dar es Salaam Hong Kong Karachi
Kuala Lumpur Madrid Melbourne Mexico City Nairobi
New Delhi Shanghai Taipei Toronto

With offices in

Argentina Austria Brazil Chile Czech Republic France Greece
Guatemala Hungary Italy Japan Poland Portugal Singapore
South Korea Switzerland Thailand Turkey Ukraine Vietnam

Oxford is a registered trade mark of Oxford University Press
in the UK and in certain other countries

Published in the United States
by Oxford University Press Inc., New York

© Oxford University Press 2009

The moral rights of the author have been asserted
Database right Oxford University Press (maker)

First published 2009

British Library Cataloguing in Publication Data

Data available

Library of Congress Cataloging in Publication Data

Data available

Typeset in Minion
by Cepha Imaging Pvt. Ltd., Bangalore, India
Printed by the MPG Books Group
in the UK

ISBN 978-0-19-923993-1 (Pbk)

10 9 8 7 6 5 4 3 2 1

Practical Patient Safety

This book is d⋯

This book is dedicated to Elaine Bromiley, victim of an unintended human error during a routine operation; and to her team of clinicians who did their best but were never given the opportunity to learn about human factors, human error and good non-technical skills until they had the lesson for real.

Preface

In 2006, Elaine Bromiley, a healthy 37-year-old woman was booked in for non-emergency sinus surgery. The theatre was very well equipped. The ENT surgeon had 30 years experience and the consultant anaesthetist had 16 years experience. Three of the four nurses in theatre were also very experienced.

Anaesthesia was induced at 8.35 a.m. but it was not possible to insert the laryngeal mask airway. By 8.37 a.m. oxygenation began to deteriorate and the patient became cyanosed. At 8.39 a.m. the oxygen saturation level had fallen to 40%. Attempts to ventilate the lungs with 100% oxygen using a facemask and oral airway proved extremely difficult. The oxygen saturation level remained perilously low and the anaesthetist who was joined by another consultant colleague was unable to perform a tracheal intubation.

By 8.45 a.m. airway access still had not been achieved and a situation existed that was termed 'can't intubate, can't ventilate'. This is a recognized emergency for which a guideline exists-to perform an emergency tracheotomy. Anticipating the need for an emergency tracheotomy, a nurse went to fetch the tracheotomy equipment. A second nurse phoned through to the intensive care unit to check there was a spare bed available.

The growing stress of the situation apparently caused the surgeon and the anaesthetists to lose awareness of how long they had been attempting to insert the tube.

The nurse who fetched the tracheotomy kit told the medical team it was available but none of the consultants subsequently recalled her speaking to them (probably due to fixation and stress). The nurse who phoned ICU addressed the consultants explaining 'There's a bed available in Intensive Care', but to quote from the Inquest they looked at her as if to say 'what's wrong? You're over-reacting.' The nurse concerned cancelled the bed with ICU, although she stated that she instinctively felt that the consultants were mis-managing the patient's care.

The three consultants decided to continue attempts at intubation, but at 9.10 a.m. they abandoned the procedure hoping that the patient would wake up. Her oxygen level remained below 40% for 20 minutes and she never regained consciousness. She died 13 days later.

If the experience of Elaine's family was an isolated one it would be tragedy enough. But it is not. Over the last few years the general public and the media have become increasingly aware of the concept of clinical error leading to patient harm. In the UK alone it has been estimated that 40 000 patients die every year as a consequence of clinical error—something their doctors or nurses did to them that led directly to their death. This is the dramatic tip of the iceberg, but below the surface lurks an even larger 'mass' of harm leading to prolonged hospital admission or permanent disability.

However one looks at it, error leading to an adverse event (patient harm) represents a failure of the system or of individuals or of both. Reflection on failure is almost always a painful exercise, but in every cloud there is a silver lining. The study of failure gives us the opportunity of learning and of avoiding failure in the future. The key is to learn from the mistakes of others. To paraphrase Bismarck: 'Only a fool learns from his own mistakes. The wise man learns from the mistakes of others.'

Unfortunately, for whatever reason, many of us, whether doctors, nurses, or hospital managers, are forced to learn from our own bitter experiences as healthcare systems are notoriously bad at translating the experience of error into preventative methods. In the foreword of the Healthcare Commission's 2006 Report into the *Clostridium difficile* outbreak at Stoke Mandeville Hospital, Sir Ian Kennedy recalled that he had *not* been able to say with confidence in the immediate aftermath of the Bristol Babies enquiry that such events would never happen again. The Stoke Mandeville experience proved his concerns to be correct and led him to state: 'It is a matter of regret that the lessons of Bristol have not been learned and incorporated into every corner of the NHS.'

Our intention in writing this book is to provide the reader with error prevention tools. These tools have been designed to incorporate the lessons learned by other unfortunate doctors and nurses who have committed errors, so that the same path towards error and adverse events can be avoided. Thus, much of the book is taken up by an analysis of accidents that have happened in healthcare and other 'industries' because we are convinced that an understanding of how error occurs is fundamental to being able to prevent error. Although human error might appear to have limitless configurations, in reality the way in which humans commit error can be distilled down to a few fundamentals. Thus, we believe that the patient safety tools described in this book can be used most effectively if the user knows how and why the tool was created in the first place.

The clinician authors have been fortunate indeed to have had the world of the airline pilot opened up to them through their co-author, Peter Stevenson. We have learnt about the techniques employed by airline pilots to enhance safety in what is potentially a high-risk environment (flying wide body passenger airliners), but which in reality is nowadays one of the safest forms of mass transportation. Such techniques are so obviously sensible, and failure to observe them so obviously central to the development of many errors that have occurred in the past in the transport, nuclear, and petrochemical industries (nowadays called high reliability organizations) that the authors believe that they should be taught to all healthcare workers as so many of the human errors of doctors and nurses mirror errors in these industries. This then is the essential purpose behind writing this book—to translate high reliability organization safety principles and techniques into the healthcare situation.

Of course, healthcare differs in several important aspects to flying aircraft. Patients are often very sick and therefore vulnerable, the 'operations' of healthcare organizations are enormously diverse and emergencies are commonplace. Added to this is the fact that, whereas the number of staff to be trained in airline safety techniques is relatively small (the ratio of aircrew to passengers numbers is very low), there is a greater balance between the numbers of patients and carers because healthcare is often delivered on a one-to-one basis—doctor to patient, nurse to patient. Thus, healthcare organizations are faced with the challenge of educating enormous numbers of doctors and nurses across a wide range of organizations and areas. Add to all this the sometimes unpredictable behaviour of patients and the potential for error on a large scale becomes obvious.

Despite these differences between planes and patients, important similarities exist between the types of errors that have occurred in the cockpits of passenger airliners, on oil rigs, on cross-channel ferries, and in the driver's cabs of passenger trains and those that occur on hospital wards and in operating theatres. These similarities relate to the fact that all these organizations rely on humans to run them and humans commit errors in a relatively limited number of ways. Aspects of human behaviour that lead to error are universal—whether the human being happens to be a pilot, a nurse, a physician, or a surgeon. Many of the safety techniques learnt by pilots and workers in other high reliability organizations relate to the way in which *human error* can be prevented. Pilots commit slips, lapses, and mistakes just as doctors do, but they are equipped with tools to help them recognize potential and evolving errors, so preventing them from occurring or mitigating their effect once they have occurred. For this reason, the safety track record of modern airlines and other high reliability organizations has improved dramatically over the last 20 years or so. The same cannot be said of healthcare.

When we talk about these techniques of error reduction, doctors sometimes say to us, 'yes, but where's the evidence?' In recent years the medical profession has (in many cases quite appropriately) become locked into the concept of evidence-based medicine, which is often founded on the principle of the randomized, controlled trial. Admirable though this may be, high reliability organizations have never felt the need for randomized controlled trials to confirm the efficacy of their safety principles. They argue that most of their safety concepts are just common sense. Airline companies regard the principle of cross-checking, for example, as critical to safe flying. They do not need to wait for the publication of a randomized trial to tell them that cross-checking that the doors of an airliner are closed is a sensible and safe thing to do. Thus, whenever you fly you will hear the expression 'doors to cross-check' as the cabin crew cross-over from one side of the aircraft to the other to confirm that the doors really are shut! Just one disaster as a consequence of a 'door closure failure' would irreparably destroy the reputation of an airline. So high reliability organizations do not feel the need to rely on an evidence base as we would understand it in the medical sense of the word. The proof for high reliability organizations lies in the common sense of the techniques they promote and their year-on-year maintenance (and often improvement) of a low incidence of errors and accidents.

During our attempts to teach medical students about the concept of error in healthcare and techniques for preventing or mitigating its effects, we are constantly asked what attempts are being instituted to make the *system* safer. As individuals working in large healthcare organizations employing many thousands of people we all suffer, from time to time, with the feeling that there is nothing we can do to change the system. It is easy to be overwhelmed by the lack of influence that the individual has in organizations that are often perceived to have low expectations for safety. This leads many to assume that error will always occur and that there is nothing they can do about it as individuals. Error experts would call this 'learned helplessness'. If there is one overriding message that we want to get across in this book, apart from the obvious message about the nuts and bolts of error prevention, it is that the *individual* doctor or nurse can *most definitely make a difference* in terms of enhancing patient safety in his or her day to day practice. They can do so by changes in behaviour that come at no cost whatsoever, other than the cost of buying and the effort of reading this book.

Most of the methods we describe do not require complex computer hardware or software. None requires weeks to be spent in a classroom, out of clinical practice. None requires vast quantities of money to be 'thrown' at the problem. What is required is the development of an *attitude* towards safety- an attitude that has become prevalent in the high reliability organizations. An attitude that error is common, that much of it is preventable and that simple techniques, as outlined in this book, can have a very substantial impact on preventing it or reducing its effects. And that attitude is an *individual* attitude (though of course strong leadership directed at patient safety should be provided within healthcare organizations so that the individual knows he or she is supported by their employer). While it is important to appreciate the in-built sources of error within the system (what James Reason, the great guru of human error analysis, would call the 'organizational' accident) so that they may be recognized, avoided, and 'designed-out' of the system, we focus principally on what Reason would call 'error wisdom' for the individual.

Inevitably there will be omissions in any book. The subject of hospital-acquired infection is an enormous one and it is beyond the scope of this book to cover this subject in the depth that it quite rightly deserves, other than to highlight the importance of preventative strategies as a way of reducing infections that often result as a consequence of error such as lapses in hand washing. For an in-depth analysis of this aspect of error the reader must consult other texts. Similarly, prescribing errors justify entire books in their own right, so we would ask the reader to forgive the limited amount of space that we have devoted to this area.

The father of modern neurosurgery, Harvey Cushing, described his great success as a neurosurgeon as having been built on a mountain of corpses. Of course not all of those patients in Cushing's mountain were there as a consequence of clinical error, but it is likely that a proportion were there because of it. While we would not describe our success as being built on a *mountain* of corpses, we are only human, and we too have committed our fair share of errors, some of which have led to patient harm. We therefore dedicate this book to all those patients who have suffered harm in our hands and at the hands of our profession in the sincere hope that in sharing our experiences and in teaching patient safety techniques, we can reduce the frequency and impact of error in healthcare.

We are not so naïve as to believe that all of the techniques and procedures described in this book will be adopted overnight by every single healthcare worker and by every single healthcare organization throughout the Western world. We know that change takes time to occur and we know that change is often met with resistance. We know that you, the individual reader will come across scepticism or surprise, indeed even ridicule, when you first start to use the techniques we describe. But persevere. We are absolutely convinced that this book contains advice that will enable you, the individual doctor or nurse, to make minor and simple changes to your day-to-day practice that will immediately translate into safer practice.

Chris Lillehei, a US surgeon, once said: 'Good judgment comes from experience; experience comes from bad judgment.'

We hope that you the reader will be able to incorporate the lessons contained in this book into your practice so that you will not need to learn from experience, but rather can develop a systematic approach to error reduction based on the experiences of others.

Note

Throughout this book the word 'man' is used in its generic sense and includes both sexes. 'He' should be understood, where appropriate, to mean 'he or she', 'his' to mean 'his/her' and so on.

Reference

Investigation into outbreaks of *C difficile* at Stoke Mandeville Hospital, Buckinghamshire Hospitals NHS Trust, July 2006. Healthcare Commission. www.healthcarecommission.org.uk

Acknowledgements

We wish to thank the following. Martin Bromiley for permission to use the case history of his late wife, Elaine. Clare Crowley, Rebecca White and Olunbunmi Fajemisin, Pharmacy Department, Oxford Radcliffe Hospitals NHS Trust for images of drug errors. Michael Murphy, Professor of Blood Transfusion Medicine, University of Oxford and Honorary Consultant Haematologist, Oxford Radcliffe Hospitals NHS Trust for advice on transfusion errors. Mr Richard Berrisford, Consultant Thoracic Surgeon, Royal Devon and Exeter Foundation NHS Trust for permission to use The Exeter Check List. Marc DeLeval, Consultant Cardiothoracic Surgeon, Great Ormond Street Hospital and the National Heart Hospital—for his inspiring studies on error in the setting of paediatric cardiothoracic surgery. Michael Woods, Head of Operations Research, Rail Safety and Standards Board for permission to use data from Report T365: Collecting and analysing railway safety critical communication error data. Tony Walton, Programme Manager, Railway Communications, Network Rail for permission to reproduce the 'Taking Lead Responsibility' advice.

Contents

Chapter 1

Clinical error: the scale of the problem

The years since the Second World War have seen enormous progress in medical science. Unfortunately, the bright light of this success had blinded doctors and nurses to a dark subject that had, until recently, been completely overlooked.

Evidence is accumulating that harm to patients resulting from errors by healthcare professionals is a very significant problem. The consequential costs in litigation, wasted time, and extra treatment create a substantial drain on the resources of healthcare systems. The resources thus wasted are unavailable for the treatment of other patients.

The Harvard Medical Practice Study[1,2] was a retrospective review of the records of over 30 000 randomly chosen patients who were admitted to 51 acute care, non-psychiatric hospitals in New York State in 1984. This study suggested that one patient in every 200 admitted to hospital died following an adverse event. This study was met with much incredulity. How could the rate of fatal adverse events be so high?

In the following years, however, further retrospective studies were carried out in six other countries, including the UK. If allowance is made for the differences in definitions used and the scope of the types of adverse events that these studies investigated, these studies confirmed that the results of the Harvard study were broadly correct. Indeed they suggested that the Harvard estimate of the frequency of adverse events was too conservative.

Across the seven different national healthcare systems 'covered' by these studies, some kind of adverse event occurred to approximately 1 in 10 hospital inpatients. Of these nearly half of all adverse events were assessed as 'preventable'. Approximately 6% of patients who suffered an adverse event were permanently disabled as a consequence of the adverse event. Approximately 8% of patients who suffered an adverse event died.

There was criticism that the retrospective study methodology was subject to bias. However, prospective studies observing clinicians at work in real time show rates of error in such activities as administering medications, communicating clinical data, blood transfusions, etc., which are of the same order as those seen in the retrospective studies.

In Britain the cost of preventable adverse events is assessed as £1 billion per annum in lost bed days alone.[3] The wider costs of lost working time, disability benefits paid to those injured by the adverse event, and the wider economic consequences add additional unmeasured costs. The Institute of Medicine report[4] estimated that, in the USA, total annual national costs (lost income, lost household production, disability, healthcare costs) were between $17 billion and $29 billion for preventable adverse events and about double that for all adverse events.

The Harvard Medical Practice Study 1984[1,2]

This study reviewed the patient records of 30 121 randomly chosen patients in 51 acute care, non-psychiatric hospitals in New York State in 1984. The goals of the study were

1. to establish the level of patient injury, and
2. to provide data for efforts to reform medical malpractice procedures.

As a consequence of the second goal only those injuries that could potentially lead to litigation (and thus represented injury due to substandard care) were measured. No attempt to detect 'near misses'—errors that did not actually harm patients—was made nor were events that caused only minor physical discomfort counted. Terminally ill patients were excluded. Thus, adverse events in patients who were certain to have died were excluded from the study.

The results

1. Adverse events occurred to 1133 (3.7%) of the 30 121 patients in the study.
2. Of these 1133 patients, 74 were 'permanently disabled' by the event.
3. 154 (0.5%) patients died following a 'clinical error'.

> This equates to 1 in 200 patients dying as a consequence of an adverse event.

Of all adverse events, 47.7% were operative events (related to surgical care) and 17% of all adverse events were deemed to have been due to negligent practice, i.e. it was judged that the management had been substandard. The most common non-operative adverse events were adverse drug events (ADEs), followed by diagnostic mishaps, therapeutic mishaps, procedure-related events, and others.

Overall, 37.2% of the non-operative events were deemed to have been due to negligent practice. As one might expect, the most common sites for adverse events were operating theatres followed by the patients' rooms, Accident and Emergency Departments, labour and delivery rooms, and ICUs.

Extrapolations from these data suggested that approximately 98 000 Americans would die each year following preventable adverse events. This would be eight times the number who die on America's roads.

The Quality in Australian Healthcare Study 1992[5]

The Quality in Australian Healthcare Study (QAHS) investigators based their study upon the Harvard methodology. However, as their goal was to gather data to improve 'quality' efforts, they were more interested in the 'preventability' of adverse events rather than 'negligence' in a medico-legal context.

They reviewed 14 179 randomly sampled records from patients in 28 hospitals in South Australia and New South Wales in 1992. As they focused on preventable events and included 'near misses' (where no harm to the patient resulted), the study uncovered a much larger number of adverse events than the Harvard study.

Using their definition of an adverse event, QAHS researchers found that 16.6% of the patients in the study experienced an adverse event. When adjusted to count adverse events according to the Harvard Study definition the rate was 13%. Of all adverse events, 51% were judged to have been preventable if there had been better communication between clinicians and better standards of checking.

The higher rates of adverse events detected in the Australian study, over four times greater than that found by the Harvard study, is partly accounted for by the wider range of adverse events included (for instance, adverse events occurring outside hospital were included), the focus on quality of care rather than negligent care, and the inclusion of many more minor events in the definition of adverse events.

As with the Harvard Study, most adverse events were related to surgical procedures (50.3%) followed by diagnostic errors (13.6%), therapeutic errors (12.0%), and ADEs (10.8%). Permanent disability resulted from 13.7% of adverse events and death from 4.9%.

> 1 in 123 patients died following a 'clinical error'.

The Australian study also found that 34.6% of errors were related to technical performance, 15.8% to a failure to synthesize and/or act upon information, 11.8% from a failure to request or arrange an investigation, procedure, or consultation, and 10.9% due to lack of care and attention or failure to attend the patient.

Communication problems between clinicians were the single most frequently occurring factors contributing to adverse incidents that harmed patients and these errors were nearly twice as common as those due to inadequate medical skill or knowledge.

The University College London Study 2001[3]

This paper announced the results of a retrospective review of the medical and nursing records of 1014 patients in two acute hospitals in the Greater London area.

The study showed that 110 (10.8%) patients experienced an adverse event, with an overall rate of adverse events of 11.7% because several patients suffered more than one event. About half of these events were judged to be preventable with ordinary standards of care. A third of adverse events led to moderate or greater disability or death. Nine patients died.

> This translated into 1 in 113 patients dying following an adverse event.

Danish, New Zealand, Canadian, and French studies

In addition to the three studies above, four others have been carried out in Denmark, New Zealand, Canada, and France. The results of all seven studies are summarized in Table 1.1. In aggregate, these latter four studies have an average adverse event rate of almost exactly 10%, which is very close to the rate in the UK UCL study.[3]

The frequency and costs of adverse drug events

One retrospective study[10] examined the frequency and cost of ADEs at the University of Virginia Hospital. The authors used an automated monitor that looked for patterns in laboratory test results and/or orders for medications that may have indicated that an ADE had taken place. For instance, if a hospital patient was prescribed naloxone (a drug used to reverse the effects of opiates), this may have indicated that the patient had received an erroneous excessive dose of morphine or other opioid. Based on an analysis of these results it was estimated that between 1996 and 1999 ADEs occurred at a rate of 10.4–11.5 adverse events per 100 admissions.

About half of these events were assessed as 'preventable errors'—roughly five events per 100 admissions. It was estimated that length of stay following a preventable ADE was extended by an average of 2.2 days per patient.

Table 1.1 The percentage of patients experiencing an adverse event (AE) in the Harvard, Australian, Danish, New Zealand, Canadian, French, and UK studies

Study	Number of hospitals (year)	Number of patient admissions	% of patients who suffered 'adverse events'	% of AEs that were 'preventable'
USA: (New York) Harvard Medical Practice Study (Brennan et al. 1991)[1]	51 (1984)	30 121	3.7 (study excluded non-preventable events)	Not assessed as the study only considered preventable events
Australia: Quality in Australian Healthcare Study (Wilson et al. 1995)[5]	28 (1992)	14 179	16.6	51.0
Denmark (Schioler et al. 2001)[6]	17 (1998)	1097	9.0	40.4
New Zealand (Davis et al. 2002)[7]	13 (1998)	6579	11.2	37.0
UK (Vincent et al. 2001)[3]	2 (1999)	1014	10.8	48.0
Canada (Baker et al. 2004)[8]	20 (2000)	3745	7.5	36.9
France (Michel et al. 2004)[9]	7 (2002)	778	14.5	Not reported

Accuracy of retrospective studies

The retrospective reviews upon which the above statistics were based, like any other research method, have their limitations and the findings of the studies have to be treated with caution because of their methodological limitations.

Graham Neale, the lead clinician in the British study, summarized the principal methodological problems, although he accepted that the level of adverse events revealed was broadly correct. Neale and Woloshynowych[11] pointed out, for instance, that the review process relies on the judgements of the doctors who reviewed the patient records.

Great efforts have been made to strengthen the accuracy and consistency of these judgements by training of observers, by the use of structured data collection, and by duplicate review.

Two factors may have an effect that might either underestimate or exaggerate the rate of adverse events in these retrospective studies.

Underestimation: failure to record erroneous acts

There is anecdotal evidence to suggest that, on occasion, doctors have chosen not to record accurately, or even at all, in the patient's medical notes an error that they have made in treating a patient. The researchers might not be able to detect such errors, although in some cases they might be inferred by subsequent treatment given to the patient. No study has attempted to gauge the extent of this underestimation problem.

Exaggeration: hindsight (outcome) bias

The principal criticism of the record review methodology used by the large-scale studies is that they may be prone to 'hindsight bias'. People tend to exaggerate in retrospect what they say they knew before an incident occurred—the 'I knew it all along' effect.

Hindsight bias might perhaps be better termed 'outcome bias'. When a clinical outcome is known to be bad, those looking back at the treatment of the patient are much more likely to be critical and more likely to define certain actions as errors. So, for example, Caplan et al.[12] asked two groups of physicians to review two sets of notes. The sets of notes were identical but one group was told that the outcomes for the patients were satisfactory and the other group was told that the outcome was poor for the patient. The group who believed the outcomes were poor made much stronger criticisms of the care, even though the care described was exactly the same. Thus we tend to simplify things in retrospect and tend to be more critical when the outcome is bad.

Kieran Walshe[13] has concluded that the recognition of adverse events by record review had moderate to good face, and validity with respect to quality of care in a hospital setting.

Error rates revealed in retrospective studies are of the same order of magnitude as those found in observational studies

The negative and positive factors described above may have the effect of balancing each other out.

Although the methodology of the retrospective studies might be criticized, it is interesting to note that on the few occasions where observational studies have been carried out on clinicians performing their duties in real time, the rates of human error observed have appeared not to be greatly different from those reported in the retrospective studies.

An as-yet-unpublished prospective study (real time observations) at the Oxford Radcliffe Hospitals Trust found that 12% of patients suffered an adverse event (Simon Kreckler, personal communication). This rate is similar to the average of the rates (10%) found by the retrospective studies in Table 1.1.

Error rates according to type of clinical activity

Communication of safety critical data over the telephone

A study by Barenfanger et al.[14] in the USA analysed the reliability of transfer of pathology laboratory results over the telephone from three pathology laboratories to doctors. These results were all urgent and in most cases the doctors would be providing immediate treatment based on the information received over the telephone. It goes without saying that it can be critical for the safe management of a patient that the *correct* result for the *correct* patient is communicated where conditions such as hyperkalaemia, or abnormal blood clotting, or a suspected myocardial infarction or pulmonary embolus is being managed. It is not too difficult to imagine that a fatal error could occur if the treating doctor bases the quantity of potassium infused into a patient on an erroneously communicated serum potassium level.

So what did Barenfenger and colleagues[14] find? 822 telephone calls from the pathology laboratories were studied. In 29 cases (3.5% of the calls) the doctor had misunderstood or mis-transcribed the data. Many of these errors had the potential to seriously endanger the patient.

Verbal communication in the operating theatre

Lingard et al.[15] reported an observational study of 42 surgical procedures in a Toronto hospital. During the 90 hours of observation there were a total of 421 verbal communications between members of the surgical team. Each communication was assessed with respect to 'occasion' (appropriate timing), 'content' (completeness and accuracy), 'purpose' (whether the message achieved its objective, or could have done), and 'audience' (whether the person addressed has the capacity to answer or whether key personnel were present).

One hundred and twenty-nine of 421 communications (30.6%) observed in the operating theatre 'failed' in one or more of these ways. Lingard et al.[15] noted that 'a third of these resulted in effects which jeopardised patient safety'. They found that 'critical information was often transferred in an ad hoc, reactive manner and tension levels were frequently high'.

Bedside blood transfusion errors

A Belgian study[16] assessed the frequency and nature of bedside transfusion errors in three hospitals in Brussels. Over a period of 15 months, 808 patients received 3485 units of blood. There were 13 serious errors (1.6% of all patients transfused), including seven cases where the patient received the wrong blood. This equates to *1 in 115 patients receiving the wrong blood*.

Checking patients prior to blood transfusions

Turner et al.[17] (National Patient Safety Agency data) analysed transfusions before and after the introduction of a bar coding system in a haematology outpatient clinic at a 1500-bed hospital in the UK. The study revealed that during the administration of blood, patients were not asked for their name in 93% of the 1500 cases, while their date of birth was not asked in 12%.

In 12% of the cases the patient was not wearing a wristband, and in 100% of the cases the patient ID on the wristband was not cross-referenced with the patient-stated ID. In 90% of the cases the special requirements on the blood pack were not cross-referenced with any requested on the prescription.

All of the checks were carried out at the bedside. During the collection of blood samples (30 observations) 43% of the patients were not asked for their name, while 50% were not asked for their date of birth; 90% of the patients were not wearing a wristband.

These statistics reflect a major and systemic failure of the checking culture.

Checking of anaesthetic machines

Mayor and Eaton[18] surveyed the checking of anaesthetic machines and showed that up to 41% of anaesthetists performed no checks on their equipment at all. This was a worrying statistic because Bartham and McClymont[19] in the same edition of *Anaesthesia* found that 18% of anaesthesia machines had 'serious faults'.

Missing test results

A number of studies have sought to establish the incidence of missed test results. Delays in diagnosis constitute a common medical error and represent a significant threat to patient safety.

An important study conducted by Roy[20] examined clinician awareness of significantly abnormal test results that had been received by the clinical team after the patient's discharge from a large teaching hospital. The investigators found that clinically important missed results occurred in nearly 1% of patient discharges.

Deaths from adverse events

> Blundering doctors 'kill 40,000 a year'

This was the main front-page headline of *The Times* newspaper on Friday 13 August 2004. The article beneath said that 'medical accidents and errors contribute to the deaths of 72,000 people a year, and they are directly blamed for 40,000.'

Media reports relating to medical accidents and errors in the USA have quoted a figure of 98 000 deaths a year there, based on the Harvard study.

The validity of these 'death rates' inferred from the Harvard and other retro-spective studies has been questioned. It has been argued, following estimates of the death rate in hospital at the time of the study, that the patients who reportedly died from adverse events in the Harvard study were already severe-ly ill and likely to die anyway.[21] In a further challenge to the figures, Hayward and Hofer[22] compared the findings with their own review of the standard of care of patients who died in hospital while having active, as opposed to pallia-tive, care. They found that only 0.5% of patients would have lived longer than 3 months even if they had all had optimal care. Thus it seems that some deaths were possibly preventable but the great majority of these people were already very ill and would have died anyway. How important an extra few months of life is deemed to be no doubt varies from person to person according to their disease and circumstances.

In a reply to McDonald *et al.*'s[21] criticisms, Lucian Leape,[23] one of the authors of the Harvard study noted that:

> Some seem to have the impression that many of the deaths attributed to adverse events were minor incidents in severely ill people. This is not so.

First terminally ill patients were excluded from the study. A review of the cases in which the care was most deficient reveals two groups of patients: a small group, 14%, who were severely ill and in whom the adverse event tipped the balance; and a larger group, 86%, for whom the error was … a major factor leading to the patient's death.

In July 2005 the National Patient Safety Agency (http://www.npsa.nhs.uk/) in the UK announced that they had received reports of 840 patient deaths following avoidable mistakes during the preceding year across the whole healthcare system (including GP's surgeries, ambulance trusts, and in community and mental healthcare). In its second report in August 2006, the agency stated that this total had risen to 2159 deaths. The higher rate in the second year undoubtedly reflects a greater level of reporting rather than a doubling of real adverse events.

Thus it seems that the true number of patient deaths from these causes lies somewhere between 2159 and 40 000.

Extra bed days as a consequence of error

The focus on the rate of patient *deaths* following adverse events has directed attention away from what is another very important consequence of clinical error.

Although 70% of patients who suffer an adverse event require no extra treatment, a small number require very prolonged treatment to recover from their adverse event. These few cases have the effect of substantially raising the overall average number of 'extra bed days'.

In one of the case studies in this book a patient who had the wrong kidney removed was judged to be unsuitable for a kidney transplant and, consequently, will require dialysis for the rest of her life. The average cost of treating a patient on hospital haemodialysis is £35 000 per year.

The UK, Danish, and Canadian studies assessed the consequences of those adverse events that had been detected in terms of the consequent extra bed days required to treat the patient. The three studies produced similar findings.

The UK study found that patients who suffer an adverse event spend, on average, an extra 8.5 days in hospital. The Danish study found an average of seven extra bed days and the Canadian six extra bed days.

In the UK study the treatment of 1014 patients was analysed. The 110 patients who suffered adverse events required a total of 999 extra bed days. Of these 460 extra bed days (46%) arose from 'preventable' events.

A rate of 460 preventable extra bed days when treating 1014 patients would equate to *every* inpatient spending, on average, almost an extra half a day in hospital recovering from a 'preventable' adverse event.

Across the NHS this would total three million extra bed days a year at a cost of at least £1 billion. Other consequential costs may add a further £1 billion per year. Clearly, preventable adverse events produce a continuing and huge drain on NHS resources.

Belief in the reliability of the adverse event rate statistics

Robinson *et al*.[24] carried out a survey in the USA of 594 doctors and 500 members of the public in order to assess the level of credence in the rates of adverse events as reported by the various studies.

> Only 21% of the doctors surveyed thought that healthcare was failing to match the safety records of other industries.

The general public was more likely than doctors to believe that the quality and safety of healthcare was a problem, that error reduction should be a priority and to support mandatory reporting of serious errors.

It appears, therefore, that a much higher proportion of the general public than of doctors is concerned about the safety of healthcare. Although the authors did not ascertain the reasons for this in their survey, they speculate that the public is unduly influenced by isolated but horrific accounts of medical errors in the media. Alternatively, they suggest, physicians do not seem to be as concerned about errors as they should be. It might be that the difficulty of defining and measuring errors and of determining their preventability has led physicians to underestimate their frequency or not to recognize them at all.

The cost to the NHS of adverse events

In November 2005 the National Audit Office in the UK issued a report into the costs of adverse events in the NHS.[25]

A total of 974 000 clinical error events per annum were officially recorded, of which half were judged preventable. This figure did not include 300 000 hospital-acquired infections, of which 30% were judged preventable. One patient in 10 suffered harm as a result of a clinical error. Of those patients who were harmed, 19% suffered 'moderate impairment', 6% suffered 'permanent impairment', and 8% died. The report also revealed that there were 2081 clinical error deaths officially recorded in the year to March 2005, although it suggested that due to a culture of under-reporting the true total could be as high as 34 000 deaths per year.

The report repeated the calculation from the UCL study[3] that the total cost of the extra bed days resulting from clinical errors is over £2 billion per year, of which one-half would be preventable.

In the year 2004–5 the NHS paid out £423 million in litigation costs. A further £50 million was paid to NHS personnel suspended on full pay during investigations into adverse events.

Criminal prosecutions for medical errors

A study reported in the *British Medical Journal*[26] showed that there had been an eightfold increase in the number of doctors charged with manslaughter during the 1990s compared with earlier decades. The report's author speculates that this might be because of 'a greater readiness to call the police or to prosecute, perhaps because the Crown Prosecution Service perceives that juries are readier to convict nowadays'.

In a later study, Ferner and McDowell[27] noted that of 85 prosecutions for manslaughter over a 20-year period, 60 (71%) were acquitted, 22 convicted, and three pleaded guilty. In 2005 there were 17 prosecutions of doctors for manslaughter in the UK. The rising trend of prosecutions continues.

Reliability: other industries

In civil aviation, European passenger railway and the nuclear power industries, the rate of catastrophic accidents in relation to the number of journeys or 'exposures' to the risk, is of the order of 1×10^6 or better.[28]

Modern passenger aircraft are, in mechanical and structural terms, extremely reliable. However, significant risks in aviation still arise from unpredictable weather conditions, congested airports and airspace, hazardous passenger behaviours, terrorism threats, and human error by pilots, controllers, and engineers. In spite of this, the national airline systems of most first world countries have, in recent years, achieved almost a 100% reliability rate (virtually zero accidents) for many consecutive years.

Reliability: healthcare

Some specialties in healthcare do achieve high levels of reliability. In anaesthetics the rate of fatal adverse events has improved markedly in the last three decades and is now approximately 1 per 100 000 anaesthetics.[28] In contrast, the rate of adverse events in surgery has been reported as 1 per 1000. Certainly, the large-scale studies carried out in the seven different nations described above do seem to confirm this rate, or suggest that it is higher still.

How high reliability organizations have been able to achieve their impressive safety records is discussed later in this book. Many of the techniques they use could very easily be translated into the healthcare setting and so doctors—and their patients—could benefit by being aware of how high reliability organizations manage to achieve high levels of reliability.

References

1 Brennan TA, Leape LL, Laird NM, *et al.* Incidence of adverse events and negligence in hospitalized patients; results from the Harvard Medical Practice Study I. *N Engl J Med* 1991; **324**: 370–6.

2 Leape LL, Brennan TA, Laird N, *et al.* The nature of adverse events in hospitalized patients. Results of the Harvard Medical Practice Study II. *N Engl J Med* 1991; **324**: 377–84.

3 Vincent C, Neale G, Woloshynowych M. Adverse events in British hospitals: preliminary retrospective record review. *Br Med J* 2001; **322**: 517–19.

4 Kohn L, Corrigan J, Donaldson ME. *To err is human.* Washington DC: National Academy Press; 1999.

5 Wilson RM, Runciman WB, Gibber RW, *et al.* The Quality in Australian Health Care Study. *Med J Aust* 1995; **163**: 458–71.

6 Schioler T, Lipczak H, Pedersen BL, *et al.* Danish adverse event study. Incidence of adverse events in hospitals. A retrospective study of medical records. *Ugeskr Laeger* 2001; **163**: 1585–6.

7 Davis P, Lay-Yee R, Briant R, *et al.* Adverse events in New Zealand public hospitals I: occurrence and impact. *N Z Med J* 2002; **115**: U271.

8 Baker GR, Norton PG, Flintoff V, *et al.* The Canadian adverse events study: the incidence of adverse events among hospital patients in Canada. *Can Med Assoc J* 2004; **170**: 1678–86.

9 Michel P, Quenon JL, de Sarasqueta AM, *et al.* Comparison of three methods for estimating rates of adverse events and rates of preventable adverse events in acute care hospitals. *Br Med J* 2004; **328**: 199.

10 Einbender JS, Scully K. Using a clinical data repository to estimate the frequency and costs of adverse drug events. *J Am Med Inform Assoc* 2002; **9**(6): S34–8.

11 Neal G, Woloshynowych M. Retrospective case record review: a blunt instrument that needs sharpening. *Qual Saf Health Care* 2003; **12**: 2–3.

12 Caplan RA, Posner KL, Cheney FW. Effect of outcome on physicians' judgments of appropriateness of care. *JAMA* 1991; **265**, 1957–60.

13 Walshe K. Adverse events in health care: issues in measurement. *Qual Health Care* 2000; **9**: 47–52.

14 Barenfanger J, Sautter RL, Lang DL *et al.* Improving patient safety by repeating ('read-back') telephone reports of critical information'. *Am J Clin Pathol* 2004; **121**: 801–3.

15 Lingard L, Espin S, Whyte S *et al.* 'Communication failures in the operating room: an observational classification of recurrent types and effects. *Qual Saf Health Care* 2004; **13**: 330–4.

16 Baele PL, De Bruyere M, Deneys V, *et al.* Bedside transfusion errors. A prospective survey by the Belgium SAnGUIS Group. *Vox Sang* 1994; **66**: 117–21.

17 Turner C, Casbard A, Murphy M. *Barcode technology: its role in increasing safety of blood transfusion* 2003. London: National Patient Safety Agency; 2003.

18 Mayor AH, Eaton JM. Anaesthetic machine checking practices. A survey. *Anaesthesia* 1992; **47**: 866–8.

19 Bartham C, McClymont W. The use of a checklist for anaesthetic machines. *Anaesthesia* 1992; **47**: 1066–9.

20 Roy CL. Patient safety concerns arising from test results that return after hospital discharge. *Ann Intern Med* 2005; **143**: 121–8.

21 McDonald CJ, Weiner M, Hui SL. Deaths due to medical errors are exaggerated in Institute of Medicine report. *JAMA* 2000; **284**: 93–5.

22 Hayward R, Hofer T. Estimating hospital deaths due medical error. *JAMA* 2001; **286**: 415–20.

23 Leape LL. Institute of Medicine medical error figures are not exaggerated. *JAMA* 2000; **284**: 95–7.

24 Robinson AR, Hohmann KB, Rifkin JI, *et al.* Physician and public opinions on quality of health care and the problem of medical errors. *Arch Intern Med* 2002; **162**: 2186–90.

25 National Audit Office/Department of Health. *A safer place for patients: learning to improve patient safety*. London: The Stationary Office; 2005.

26 Ferner R. Medication errors that have led to manslaughter charges *Br Med J* 2000; **321**: 1212–16.

27 Ferner RE, McDowell SE. Doctors charged with manslaughter in the course of medical practice. *J R Soc Med* 2006; **99**: 309–14.

28 Amalberti R, Auroy Y, Berwick D, Barach P. Five system barriers to achieving ultrasafe health care, *Ann Intern Med* 2005; **142**(9): 756–64.

Chapter 2

Clinical errors: What are they?

In this chapter we describe generic types of clinical errors that can occur in day-to-day practice together with practical ways of preventing these common sources of error. By generic we mean those errors that are common to many, if not all specialties and all areas of practice. We are certain that our list of errors is neither comprehensive nor exhaustive, for there is an almost limitless number of ways in which humans can err. However, we believe the errors we describe occur commonly.

We have identified potential sources of error along the so-called patient pathway—the route that patients take from consulting their primary care doctor and then onwards through the hospital system. This pathway is one that is familiar to every doctor and so we hope that it will allow sites of error to be put into the context of day-to-day practice. Thinking about error in this way requires no complex classification system, but simply describes errors that can happen as the patient passes from the clinic consultation, through the process of investigation and from there to admission, operation (for surgical specialties), postoperative care, and subsequent discharge. At multiple points along this pathway errors are waiting to catch out the unwary.

The specific errors of wrong site and side surgery are discussed in Chapters 6 and 7 and are mentioned here only in passing.

Sources of error in primary care and office practice

Systematic studies of error in primary care and office-based practice in the medical and surgical specialties are few. This is unfortunate, as the bulk of care in most healthcare systems is delivered in the primary care situation. Wilson and Sheikh[1] found only 31 articles of direct relevance to error and error prevention in primary care over a period of 20 years. Most reported errors have been those related to prescribing drugs.

In the setting of primary care, Makeham *et al.*[2] have identified errors relating to the processes of healthcare as being more common (70% of errors) than those relating to deficiencies in knowledge and skills of health professionals (30%). More specifically, 12% of errors involved a diagnostic error, 20% of errors related to the prescribing of medications, and 13% involved communication problems.

As much clinical error is generic many hospital-based errors will also be of relevance to those working in primary care. The same errors of misidentification, in note-keeping, diagnosis, and prescribing occur whether you practice in primary care or in hospital and so we hope the primary care practitioner will find the rest of this chapter useful.

Sources of error along the patient pathway in hospital care and potential methods of error prevention

The path that a patient takes in their journey through a hospital starts either with the receipt of a letter of referral from the patient's primary care practitioner or as a consequence of self-referral to a hospital Emergency Department.

> Generic errors (common to primary care and hospital-based practice) can occur at key points in the patient pathway. Knowledge of these error points allows the *individual* doctor to take preventative action, thereby mitigating the effects of systems errors.

Errors in dealing with referral letters

These include:

- failure to read the letter in a timely fashion
- failure of the letter to be read by someone who understands the significance of its contents
- failure to read the whole letter
- framing errors.

Failure to 'manage' referral letters appropriately are not uncommon sources of error. Act appropriately when the referral letter arrives. Delay in dealing with the problem contained therein could lead to harm. The letter should be read by someone of sufficient seniority who is able to make informed judgements concerning the urgency of the referral.

It seems so obvious to say read the referral letter all the way to the bottom line, but this is important because relevant information may be hidden in the 'depths' of the letter and without reading the letter all the way to the end, an error in prioritizing the urgency with which the case should be dealt with may occur.

The concept of 'framing' errors is discussed later, but briefly this is where an assumption is made by the referring doctor about the significance of the presenting symptoms, with a tendency to downplay their true significance. The danger is that the investigating doctor may be so influenced by the way in which the referral letter is phrased, that he may underinvestigate important symptoms, rather than taking the symptoms at face value. So, for example, in a patient referred with macroscopic haematuria the referral letter might read something like: '… he has had several episodes of blood in his urine over the last few months and on each occasion nothing has come of it. The bleeding always stops and I suspect there is nothing going on. Can I take it that there is no need for me to refer him to you?' The referring doctor has assumed that because the previous episodes resolved spontaneously, the current episode will probably do the same. He assumes that the spontaneous resolution of the bleeding implies that there is no serious underlying cause. His referral letter is *framed* in such a way as to downplay the significance of the symptoms. The danger is that the investigating doctor may be lured into thinking in the same way. However, we know that bladder and kidney cancers bleed *intermittently*; the bleeding usually resolves spontaneously and this is often taken to imply that there cannot be any serious cause for the problem. Nothing could be further from the truth. All the while that investigation is delayed the bladder or kidney cancer is relentlessly progressing towards an advanced stage.

Errors of identification

These errors are legion! They include:

- speaking to the wrong patient
- performing procedures on the wrong patient (X-rays, blood tests, operations)
- mislabelling of blood and other pathological specimens (putting the wrong patient identification label on the specimen bottle)
- failure to label blood and other pathological specimens
- speaking to the wrong relatives
- operating on the wrong person.

Once the patient arrives at the hospital, one of the first errors that may occur (either on the first or on any subsequent interaction with healthcare workers) is an error of identification—thinking you are talking to Mr Jones when in fact you are actually addressing Mr Smith. Anecdotal evidence (the combined authors' own experiences over 50 cumulative years of clinical practice) suggests that these are *very* common sources of error. Failure to *actively* identify patients can occur at multiple points along the patient pathway:

- Getting the wrong patient into the consulting room
- Looking at a pathology report or radiology images of a different patient to the one in front of you (e.g. the wrong patient's reports may be filed in the notes). An audit of 500 sets of patients notes in our own hospital found that this occurred in about 10% of patients' notes. We were staggered to discover this.

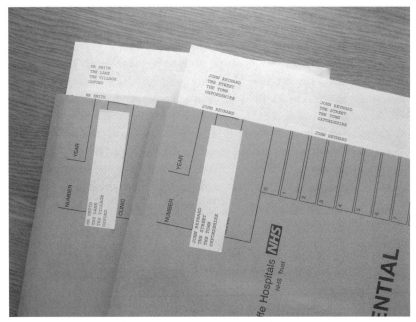

Fig. 2.1 Addressogram labels for a Mr Reynard and Mr Smith.

◆ Sticking another patient's 'addressogram' label on a pathology specimen bottle or x-ray request form of the relevant patient ('addressograms' are sticky labels kept in the notes and used for labelling investigation request forms or admission forms). In the same audit of notes, we found that the addressogram labels of another patient were filed in the wrong patient's notes in 1% of notes—so it is uncommon, but it most certainly does occur (Figs 2.1 and 2.2).

◆ Operating on the wrong patient.

At best these errors can be very embarrassing for the healthcare worker who commits them; at worst, the wrong patient can undergo an inappropriate operation. In some cases serious harm has occurred.

Errors of identification (misidentification) are a very common source of error.

Getting the wrong patient into the consulting room

Many patients are elderly and deaf or have impaired hearing. In the UK, the Royal National Institute for Deaf People (RNID), estimates that 1 in 7 adults are hard of hearing. Not surprisingly, in the setting of an outpatient clinic,

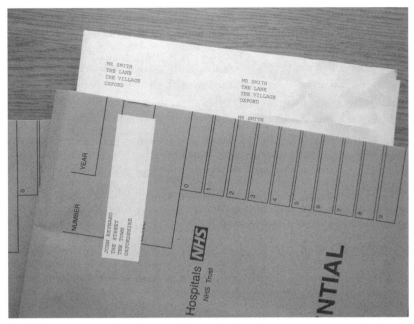

Fig. 2.2 It is surprisingly easy for another patient's addressogram labels to 'find' there way into another patient's notes. This simple error of filing can have disastrous consequences.

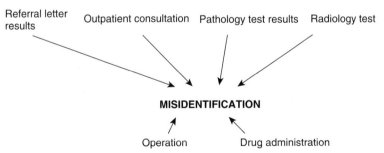

Fig. 2.3 There are multiple points along the patient pathway at which misidentification can occur. These errors are very common and are entirely preventable by the application of very simple rules.

for example, or a radiology department, patients sometimes mistakenly think you have called their name, when in fact you called the name of another patient.

There have been instances where the wrong patient enters the consulting room, is told they have cancer and then is very upset when it becomes apparent that they are not the patient you thought you were talking to! It is surprising how often this happens and it is entirely avoidable by 'active' identification.

A version of the following really did take place. The scene is a surgical outpatient consultation. Mr Smith is called into the consulting room. There are two Mr Smiths present in clinic today (hardly surprising—it is a common name) and they just happen to have similar appointment times. The correct Mr Smith pops out to the toilet at the very time that the doctor is due to call him into the room. The wrong Mr Smith hears his name being called and enters the consulting room.

The doctor does not actively identify the patient, by asking the patient to confirm his date of birth and address, and by cross-referencing this to the referral letter and notes. He simply assumes that the Mr Smith in front of him is the man who had a colonoscopic biopsy a week ago.

The following exchange of words is typical.

Doctor: 'Mr Smith, I'm sorry to have to tell you, but the biopsy of your colon shows that you have an aggressive bowel cancer and unfortunately the CT scan shows that this cancer has spread to your liver …'.

Mr Smith looks surprised. The doctor takes his surprised expression to indicate his shock at being given the bad news. The doctor continues:

Doctor: 'The spread to the liver means that we cannot cure the cancer … it also means that I'm afraid that your prognosis is not good …'.

At this point the patient interrupts the doctor.

Mr Smith: 'But doctor, I've never had a biopsy of the colon.'

Doctor: 'What do you mean, I've got the result here in front of me?'

Mr Smith: 'I'm telling you, I've never had a colon biopsy.'

And then the penny drops!

Doctor: 'Ah … are you Mr John Smith?'

Mr Smith: 'No, I'm Mr Peter Smith …'.

Oh dear! Fortunately no harm has been done, other than to the doctor's reputation. The doctor looks completely stupid. The patient may shrug this off, but his confidence in the doctor's general ability to manage patients has probably taken a turn for the worse. After all, the patient could hardly be blamed for thinking 'If the doctor can't get the right patient into the room, how can I be sure he'll check that he's operating on the right patient?'

How to avoid this error

In a phrase, use active identification. It is that simple!

> Mr Smith, could you just confirm your date of birth and address.

Its pretty unlikely that there will be two completely unrelated Mr Smith's with the same date of birth living at the same address who just happen to turn up to the clinic today, completely independently of each other. Possible, but highly unlikely.

When confirming patient identity, do not do so by reading the address and date of birth to the patient. For the same reason (deafness, for example) that they misheard the wrong name in the first place, they may not hear the address you read to them and a nod or 'yes' is not necessarily proof that they are who you think they are.

Getting the patient's address wrong

Over a 10-year period when one of the authors was a medical student and then a junior doctor training in various surgical specialties in various hospitals, he moved address on no fewer than eight occasions. Similarly, patients move house from time to time. Addressograms referring to the old address often remain in the patient's notes. Nobody takes responsibility for removing the old address labels and as a consequence (and because the doctor fails to actively identify the patient's address), the correspondence relating to the patient's booked operation or radiological investigation goes to an old address. The potential for important letters to go astray, or for notification about important investigations or operations to be sent to the wrong address, is easy to see. Delays that may impact on the patient's well being may occur.

Thus, the process of active identification serves an additional function—it allows you to double check that all correspondence relating to the patient's further investigations or treatment goes to the correct address.

It is true that doctors are not filing clerks, but if they find old addressogram labels in the notes, they are ideally positioned to prevent future errors from occurring, by simply throwing the old labels away. Try to avoid the 'it's not my job' mentality. You might argue that you are a terribly important surgeon or physician—and well you might be. However, all your brilliant diagnostic or operative skills may go to waste if an important test is delayed and the cancer or other serious condition is not diagnosed and treated when at an early, potentially curable, or reversible stage. Make it your job to 'cleanse' hospital notes of old addressograms.

The wrong addressogram labels in the patient's notes

From time to time, the wrong patient's addressograms are filed in the notes of the patient in front of you. As stated above, this occurs in about 1% of notes in our hospital. That this might occur seems so unlikely, but the following error really did occur in our own hospital.

The prostate biopsy clinic is busy. You are behind schedule. You take a biopsy from Mr Jones and stick an addressogram label on the formalin-containing specimen bottle and you make a note in Mr Jones' notes of the details of the biopsy. You don't bother to look at the addressogram labels. After all, how could the wrong labels *possibly* get into the wrong set of notes? Surely this just couldn't happen. Or could it?

When a histology report comes back on a Mr Peters, you ask to review his notes. You cannot find any evidence in Mr Peters' notes that he ever had a prostate biopsy. How strange! You go back to the list of patient's that you biopsied on that particular day. No patient called Mr Peters had a biopsy on that date, or for that matter at any point this year. You start to worry. This is all the more concerning because the pathology report suggests that 'Mr Peters', whoever he is, has a high-grade prostate cancer, which will need treatment.

Later that week, Mr Jones turns up to clinic to receive the results of the prostate biopsy. He is anxious. He found the whole process of the biopsy very painful and he is concerned about the possible diagnosis of prostate cancer. Unfortunately, no biopsy result on Mr Jones can be found. Your description of the biopsy procedure is clearly written in his notes and yet there is no report on the computer. You double check that you've got the correct Mr Jones in front of you and indeed you have. However, despite your calls to the lab, no pathology result can be found.

During your vain search through Mr Jones' notes, you find a sheet of addressogram labels on a Mr Peters filed in the back of Mr Jones' notes. Now the penny drops. You have put one of Mr Peters' addressogram labels on Mr Jones' biopsy specimen bottle!

The pathology department refuses to reissue a pathology report. As far as the pathologists are concerned the specimen they received was from Mr Peters and they must stand by the report. You now have to tell Mr Jones that you will have to do another set of biopsies. He is not going to be happy!

How on earth could this have happened you think? How on earth could the wrong identification labels have got into Mr Jones' notes? Any of 30 or so staff on the ward or in the clinic could have filed the wrong addressogram labels in Mr Jones' notes (or indeed any number of staff who over the years have come into contact with Mr Peters' and Mr Jones' notes could have filed the wrong addressograms in the wrong set of notes. Presumably at some stage their notes have been in close proximity at the same time and in the same place). It will be impossible to find the 'guilty' person (if the subsequent investigation indulges in a 'blame' approach to error causation), but what will be obvious to all concerned during the subsequent investigation is that *you* stuck the wrong label on the biopsy specimen bottle. It just isn't fair, you think. You and the patient have been the last unfortunate victims in an error chain. What is obvious is that you have been set up by a system that allows such an error to occur!

It is difficult to know how wrong addressogram filing can be prevented. It should not happen of course, but from time to time the wrong labels will inadvertently find their way into the wrong set of notes. What is clear though, is that, although such errors really do occur, you, the individual doctor, can prevent an adverse event materializing by double checking that the addressogram labels match the patient and the notes in front of you.

Exactly the same error can occur in the context of blood tests or X-ray request forms. So the lesson is clear. Whenever you request an investigation or do a procedure that requires the taking of a specimen from a patient (biopsy, blood, etc), make sure you look at the addressogram label to ensure that the label you put on the specimen bottle refers to the patient in front of you.

We now make a habit of actively identifying all patients as they walk into the consultation room, by asking them to give their date of birth and to confirm their address. We then remove any old addressogram labels from the notes and throw them away. Then, and only then, the consultation can start.

Looking at the wrong pathology or radiology results

Just as addressogram labels can be filed in the wrong set of notes, occasionally so too can the results of blood and urine tests. How often this occurs we do not know, but we think that we see an example of this on at least a monthly basis. The paper system of filing results on pathology mount sheets that have adhesive strips to which pathology reports are stuck, seems to be designed to make it as difficult as possible to see the name and other identifying features of the patient to whom they refer. Electronic case records, when they are introduced in your hospital (and in some cases the 'when' could be some time off) should eliminate many of these problems.

It is not too difficult to access the wrong patient's radiology or pathology test results on the computer systems that nowadays store radiology and pathology results. Many patients have very similar names. With the old system of storage of X-rays from time to time the wrong X-rays were filed in the wrong X-ray packet.

Occasionally you may inadvertently pick up a set of notes that do not correspond to the patient you are dealing with. Check the name—and also the

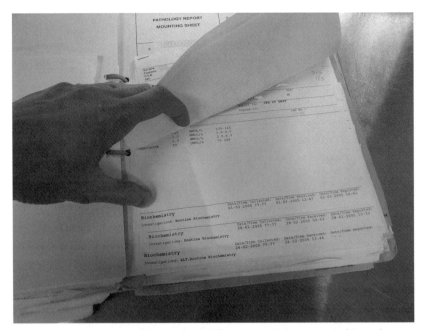

Fig. 2.4 Pathology mount sheets make it difficult to read the name and record number of the patient to whom they (supposedly) refer. The real identity of the patient may be hidden. Make sure you check that the name of the patient at the *top* of the pathology report really is that of the patient you think you are dealing with.

date—of investigations and cross-reference these against the identity of the patient you are dealing with.

The wrong patient details on dictated letters

As I write this, I am reminded of a letter that I dictated a few weeks ago, that was returned to me for signing. I remember the details of the case well and the consultation was fresh in my memory. The name and address of the patient on the head of the letter was, however, completely wrong. As luck would have it, the name on the letter was so unusual a name that I remember having never met anybody that was so-named. In addition, the patient's date of birth indicated that they were 102 years old. Having met a patient of this age would have impressed me, but I had certainly not met a 102-year-old woman that month. The secretary who had typed the letter made a seemingly minor error, in putting the wrong patient's name at the head of the letter.

Had I not spotted the error, at best, the patient receiving it would have been very confused. Importantly, from a safety perspective, safety critical information contained within the letter would not have been filed in the correct patient's notes. This has all sorts of patient safety connotations.

Operating on the wrong patient

Wrong site and wrong side surgery is relatively uncommon, but is devastating for patient and surgeon alike (obviously more devastating for the patient!). In Chapter 7 ('Situation awareness'), an example of a near miss wrong side operation is described. The incidence and causes of wrong site surgery are discussed in detail in Chapter 7, along with preventative techniques.

How to avoid errors of identification

So, errors of misidentification are common. How can they be prevented?

Confirm the patient's identity by cross-checking against at least one, and preferably two, other sources of information relating to the patient. In the context of a surgical operation, ideally you should do this *before* the patient is anaesthetized, in the anaesthetic room. In the context of some other interventional procedure such as gastroscopy, colonscopy, liver biopsy, etc., simply ask the patient to confirm their date of birth and address, while you hold their notes and check from written entries and radiology or pathology reports that the patient in front of you really is who you think it is. In the context of giving the patient a dose of some medication, simply ask the patient to confirm their date of birth and address and confirm this against their date of birth and address as written on their drug chart.

It's that simple! However, it must be done for *every* such interaction between you, the doctor or nurse and the patient and because there are so many, many interactions if we do not adhere to this rule, we will from time to time, operate on the wrong patient or give the wrong patient a drug not intended for them.

Identification of the correct patient is crucial to any activity that involves referring to a patient's notes, a pathology or radiology test result, an operation or the administration of a drug. A 'drug' can be a pharmaceutical agent, a blood product, or intravenous fluid, etc.

You may think that all these possible scenarios of identification errors are rare or couldn't possibly happen to you. Nothing could be further from the truth. Some of the most senior, most respected physicians and surgeons we know have committed identification errors!

Avoid errors of identification by active identification. Ask the patient to confirm their address and date of birth and cross-check their answer with their notes.

Errors in note keeping

The doctor's poor handwriting (and by inference poor note keeping) used to be a bit of a joke. Doctors were renowned for their illegible written notes. In the era of healthcare error, the old joke has turned somewhat sour. Poor handwriting and the broader problem of poor note keeping are a common source of error. A simple error of handwriting—mistaking an 'R' for an 'L' or a misplaced decimal point so a drug dose is wrong by a factor of 10—can and has, led to serious patient harm or death.

If your handwriting is illegible, slow down or use capitals. Time and date any clinical entries in the notes and clearly identify your name, who you are and what position you hold ('John Reynard, Consultant Urologist'). Write down your bleep or pager number or mobile phone number so you can be easily contacted if need be.

In the UK, the General Medical Council specifies that doctors should: 'keep clear, accurate, legible and contemporaneous records which report the clinical findings, the decisions made, the information given to patients and any drugs or treatment prescribed'.[3] The Royal College of Surgeons of England (RCS)[4] and the Royal College of Physicians make similar recommendations, and they do so because errors in note keeping are not infrequently an important factor in the generation of error.

Errors with medical records in general

Beware the patient with multiple sets of notes. That a patient might have several sets of notes is hardly surprising. Patients have often attended more than one specialist department. Those with chronic illnesses can generate thick sets of notes within the space of a few years. Patients who attend the Emergency Department often have temporary sets of notes made up, which eventually metamorphose into a full (non-temporary) set or are combined with their existing main set of notes (that is the theory—in practice it seems, to this author at least, that temporary sets of notes often remain as such).

Inefficient central medical records departments may fail to retrieve notes for a clinic attendance and specialist departments sometimes try to get round the problem by holding their own case records separate from the main record. A diabetic patient with chronic bronchitis could well have three sets of notes (main record, diabetes clinic, and chest clinic)—held separately and with no cross-referencing. This practice is potentially dangerous, but widespread. Electronic case records should eliminate the problem.

None of this would be a problem if it were clear from the front of the notes that the set you were holding happened to be volume 2 of three sets. Then you would know that some vital, safety critical piece of information might be contained in volumes 1 and 3, but not in set 2 (a relevant, previous adverse event, for example). The problem is that there may be no reference on the front of the notes that a patient has two or more sets of notes. Several times a month I come across examples like this, where none of the sets is a full record of the patient's medical history, investigations, or treatment, and there is absolutely no reference whatsoever that multiple sets relevant to that patient exist.

Other slips in letters that you have dictated

Secretaries, like doctors, are only human. From time to time they make mistakes. Omission of a single word such as 'not' from a letter, or substitution of 'right' for 'left' can sometimes change the meaning of the letter. So, read what you *think* you have written to ensure that there are no errors (Fig. 2.5). This is tedious, but important. Nothing may come of the error, but occasionally it can be the catalyst for the development of a serious adverse event.

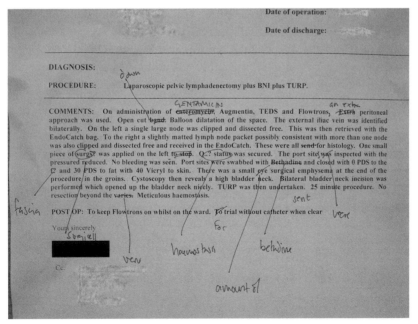

Fig. 2.5 When dictating letters read what you *think* you have written to ensure that there are no errors. This is an extreme example of a letter full of errors.

Errors as a consequence of patients failing to attend appointments for investigations or for outpatient consultations

A substantial number of patients fail to attend outpatient appointments. In some hospitals these are known as 'DNAs' ('did not arrive' or 'did not attend'). Similarly, some patients fail to attend for important investigations such as flexible cystoscopies or radiological tests during their 'work-up' for the symptom of haematuria, for example. As a substantial proportion of patients with haematuria have urological cancers, which if diagnosed early enough can be cured, then failure to attend for these investigations can cause a delay in diagnosis and subsequent treatment.

The response to such DNAs is variable. Some surgeons send another appointment and if the patient fails to attend this appointment no others are made. So-called 'DNA' letters are variable in content and most seem to be written to the patient's GP and not to the patient. They often state 'your patient failed to attend a second outpatient appointment. I have not made another one'. Presumably the surgeon expects the GP to contact the patient and admonish them.

All of this represents poor communication. It is possible that the patient has not appreciated the potential significance of their symptoms. If you don't tell a patient that macroscopic haematuria may be due to a cancer in their bladder or kidney, they may assume that its resolution indicates that the problem has gone away.

Send a DNA letter directly to the patient, with a copy to the GP. Explain in the letter why it is so important that they attend for follow-up. Be explicit. If you do not mention the possibility that the patient may have an undiagnosed cancer, you are not giving them adequate information.

If the patient fails to attend a second time, write a second letter warning them of the possible consequences of failing to attend. Lawyers talk about so-called 'contributory negligence'. The patient may contribute to a delay in the diagnosis of their cancer by failing to attend an outpatient clinic or radiological investigation. However, the doctor may also contribute by not communicating to the patient the significance of failing to attend. A lawyer may argue that a single DNA letter to a patent, or one that is vaguely worded (rather than specifically mentioning the possibility of a missed diagnosis of cancer, for example) is not enough. Avoid contributing to the negligence by making a big effort to warn the patient of the implications of their actions or, as the case may be, their inactions.

Washing your hands between patients and attention to infection control

The subject of hospital hygiene is a huge one and it is beyond the scope of this book to discuss all aspects of prevention of healthcare or hospital-acquired infections (HAI). However, it is obligatory for every healthcare worker to receive infection control training and for them to be familiar with local and national guidance. There is no excuse for cutting corners or for sloppy behaviour. In April 2008 with the enactment of the Corporate Manslaughter Act the law changed and we shall no doubt soon see prosecutions for corporate manslaughter in cases of fatal HAI.

Healthcare-associated infection

Effective prevention and control of Healthcare Associated Infections has to be embedded into everyday practice and applied consistently by everyone

The Health Act 2006 Code of Practice for Prevention and Control of Healthcare Associated Infections[5]

In 2006 a prevalence study estimated that 8.2% of inpatients in England had acquired a healthcare-associated infection of some sort.[6] In recent years, attention has focused on infections due to MRSA and *Clostridium difficile* and a number of very high-profile outbreaks have occurred. It is difficult to calculate the overall burden of HAI because it is usually not the sole cause of morbidity and mortality. However, the National Audit Office calculated in 2000[7] that HAI cost the NHS £1 billion each year. It is clear from death certification records that both MRSA and *C. difficile* contribute to many thousands of deaths every year in the UK and it is a Government and NHS priority to reduce HAI.

HAI is one of the most significant threats to patient safety and one of the biggest concerns patients have when coming into hospital. Why are hospitals such hazardous places? First, concentrating patients within a single area enhances exposure to infective agents. Secondly, inpatients have higher rates of intrinsic risk factors for acquiring infection—they are more likely to be elderly, have multiple pathologies, and are subject to invasive procedures. Finally, antibiotic usage is common—about 30% of all inpatients will be receiving an antibiotic at any one time.

Despite the frequency with which HAI occurs, there is a relative dearth of high-quality evidence on which to base guidance for reducing the burden of disease. The Department of Health *Saving Lives: reducing infection, delivering clean and safe care* document[6] focuses on 'care bundles'—drawn from the latest evidence available. This provides a way for healthcare organizations and individual practitioners to reduce the incidence of HAI.

Consider the following case:

An 84-year-old woman is admitted to an elderly care ward because she has become unsteady on her feet and is mildly confused. She has well controlled heart failure, type II diabetes, and polymyalgia rheumatica. An initial assessment finds no clear pointers for her deterioration but a urine dipstick is positive and so an MSU is sent and she is commenced on intravenous cefuroxime for a presumed urinary infection. Three days later on a Friday, the MSU reveals no significant growth and she is no better. The antibiotics are not reviewed over the weekend and she remains on them until the consultant ward round on Tuesday morning. There is a suspicion she may in fact have had a small cerebrovascular event and gradually she begins to improve. Five days later she is again unwell and 2 days later develops diarrhoea. A stool sample is sent and the next day *C. difficile* toxin is identified and she commences on treatment in accordance with local guidelines. Despite this she develops fulminant colitis and dies.

This patient was at high risk for HAI, being elderly and having multiple pathologies. Unfortunately, she was managed inappropriately on a number of fronts. First, she was given antibiotics when none was indicated—positive dipstick tests in the absence of urinary symptoms should not prompt treatment, as asymptomatic bacteriuria is common in elderly women. The antibiotics used were inappropriately broad spectrum, she did not require intravenous treatment, and they were given for too long. No one reviewed her treatment in the light of the MSU results. The diagnosis of *C. difficile* infection was not contemplated early enough and there was delay in initiating treatment while the laboratory processed the stool sample.

Paying attention to antimicrobial prescribing ('antibiotic stewardship') is central to reducing HAI and all Trusts are required to implement policies and guidelines to reduce overprescribing and inappropriate antibiotic usage. Ensure that you know how to access your local Trust guidelines and that you prescribe responsibly.

Whenever you contemplate an invasive procedure you must be able to justify it. Does this patient need a peripheral cannula? Few, if any, people come to harm from lack of a 'just in case' peripheral line, whereas MRSA bacteraemia is strongly associated with the presence of cannulae.

If you are inserting a peripheral line always follow best practice guidelines:[6]

Insertion

- *Hand hygiene*—decontaminate
- *Personal protective equipment*—gloves and if necessary gowns/aprons
- *Skin preparation*—alcohol or chlorhexidine in alcohol

- *Dressing*—sterile, semipermeable, and transparent
- *Documentation*—record date of insertion in the notes.

Ongoing care

- *Hand hygiene*—decontaminate
- *Continuing clinical indication*—is it still absolutely necessary?
- *Site inspection*—at least daily inspection for inflammation/infection
- *Dressing*—intact dry adherent dressing
- *Cannula access*—alcohol or chlorhexidine in alcohol before accessing the cannula
- *Administration set replacement*—after administration of blood products
- *Routine cannula replacement*—aim to replace within 72 hours.

There are other care bundles covering insertion of central venous and dialysis catheters and urinary catheters with which you should also be familiar.

If a patient is in a side room because they have suspected or proven infection do not enter the room without gowning up, decontaminating your hands and using gloves. Medical students in particular seem to believe they are bacteria-free zones and that by standing silently at the back of a room they are somehow exempt from passing on infection. Many Trusts have a no white coat, no tie, and 'bare below the elbow policy' when working in clinical areas and even the most senior consultant should adhere to this and set a good example.

Handwashing

It goes without saying that washing your hands before and after any patient contact is a critical aspect of patient safety. Handwashing can have a very significant impact on reducing transmission of infectious diseases such as MRSA and *C. difficile*. The father of modern surgery, Lord Lister worked this out in the 1860s. So too did Semmelweiss, an obstetrician working in Vienna in the 1850s who noted a reduced puerperal sepsis rate when medical students washed their hands after dissecting bodies in the dissection room and before delivering babies on the maternity ward. Interestingly, there was huge scepticism at the time that handwashing could be such an effective method of reducing the spread of infection.

Thus, there is nothing new in the concept that handwashing reduces the spread of infection, but it is a message that has, until recently, taken a backstage in our excitement over high technology solutions to disease such as multi-million pound MRI (magnetic resonance imaging) scanners, and the sequencing of the human genome. These latter developments hold enormous potential for the diagnosis and treatment of disease, but we should not forget the very simple techniques that can have an equally big impact.

> Handwashing between any patient contact reduces the spread of infectious diseases, such as MRSA and *Cl. difficile.*

Admission to hospital

* *Prevention of mis-identification errors.* It is now common practice for patients to wear two identification bracelets when admitted to hospital. In days gone by the single identification label was sometimes cut off to allow insertion of an intravenous line into the arm. The unconscious patient was then left without any source of identification!

* *Prevention of venous thromboembolic disease (VTE).* A recent House of Commons Select Committee has reported that a substantial number of hospitalized patients, many of them undergoing surgery, do not receive measures to prevent deep vein thrombosis (DVT) and pulmonary emboli and then subsequently develop a DVT or pulmonary embolism.[8] We sometimes think that most people who develop VTE in hospital are patients who have undergone surgery. In fact, most hospitalized patients who die from VTE are medical patients who have received inadequate VTE prophylaxis.[9] Mortality from VTE after hospital admission is at least 10 times greater than that due to MRSA. Data from post mortems indicates that 10% of deaths in hospital are due to pulmonary embolism,[9] although many of these are agonal events in terminally ill patients in whom thromboprophylaxis may have been deemed inappropriate.

When writing up a patient's medication, remember to write 'TED stockings' on the prescription chart and if they have additional risk factors for VTE, consider prescribing a low molecular weight heparin (see Table 2.1).

The use of VTE prophylaxis is discussed in further detail below.

Attention to detail in just these two areas could have a substantial impact on enhancing patient safety.

Diagnostic errors in general

Most of the literature relating to medical error focuses on events that arise after a diagnosis has been reached, i.e. on the formulation and implementation of a treatment plan. It is much harder to quantify the scale of harm that arises during the diagnostic process itself—from inadequacy of information gathering, misinterpretation of information, ignorance, inexperience,

Table 2.1 Recommended deep vein thrombosis (DVT) prophylaxis relative to risk category for patients undergoing surgical procedures

Risk category	Recommended DVT prophylaxis
Low risk: minor* surgery, <40 years old, no additional risk factors†	Elastic thromboembolism stockings for minor open surgery (none needed for minor endoscopic surgery)
Moderate risk: minor or major* surgery in patients aged 40–60 years with no additional risk factors or major surgery, <40 years old with no additional risk factors or minor surgery in those with additional risk factors	Elastic thromboembolism stockings *or* subcutaneous heparin 2 hours pre-operatively* *or* intermittent pneumatic compression stockings
High risk: Major surgery in patients >60 years old or major surgery in patients aged 40–60 with additional risk factors	Elastic thromboembolism stockings + subcutaneous heparin 2 hours pre-operatively* *or* interittent pneumatic compression stockings

*Minor surgery is defined by these guidelines as any procedure taking less than 30 minutes and major surgery as any procedure taking more than 30 minutes.

†Additional risk factors include any of the following—diagnosis of cancer, previous DVT or pulmonary embolism, obesity, varicose veins, heart failure, oestrogen use (including HRT), hypercoagulable states.

and poor judgement. Daily experience tells us that the process of formulating a diagnosis and subsequent management plan is likely to be a highly complex and error-prone process. In both the Harvard Medical Practice Study and the Quality in Australian Healthcare Study, diagnostic errors formed a significant proportion of preventable medical mishap.

Take the following common clinical example:

An 82-year-old woman with reduced mobility due to osteoarthritis goes to her GP because she has been gradually gaining weight and is a bit breathless. The GP makes a diagnosis of cardiac failure based on her account of increased breathlessness and the observation that she has swollen ankles. He thinks her jugular venous pressure may be elevated but was 'never very good at JVPs'. An open access echocardiogram, ECG, and some blood tests are requested in accordance with the local guidelines and in the meantime he issues a prescription for furosemide 40 mg and arranges to see her again in a week when he will consider adding in an ACE (angiotensin-converting enzyme) inhibitor. Five days later, before her investigations are available, the woman suffers a fall at home caused by postural hypotension while getting up too quickly from her chair because she was rushing to the toilet. She fractures her hip and dies of pneumonia 8 days after surgery.

The doctor is unaware that any of his actions may have contributed to his patient's death and assumes it is entirely in keeping with the known high mortality rate following the fractured neck of the femur in frail elderly patients with heart disease. However, where may he have failed his patient in this apparently straightforward 10-minute consultation?

- Did he take an adequate history? Had she in fact gained weight because of reduced mobility and her breathlessness is secondary to weight gain and difficulty in walking?
- Did he perform an adequate examination?
- The interpretation of her physical signs was poor. Proper assessment of the jugular venous pressure is not always easy and is subject to significant inaccuracy (the accuracy of physicians identifying an elevated jugular venous pressure was only 60% in one recent study[10]).
- He didn't consider an alternative diagnosis. Was the ankle oedema due to chronic venous disease and immobility?
- He had a busy clinic and maybe he did not spend enough time establishing the facts and coming to a decision.
- He seems to have been very keen to start drug treatment despite a lack of immediate clinical urgency to prescribe. Did she really need treatment before the results of the investigations were available?
- He prescribed a loop diuretic in a patient with reduced mobility living alone who was not acutely unwell and arguably failed to risk-assess his decision.

This clinical scenario is typical of many played out across the country every day and serves to underline the importance of paying attention to detail. Making a diagnosis can be blindingly easy when experience and pattern recognition tells you straight away what you are dealing with; however, in many areas of medicine reaching an accurate diagnosis is an iterative process spread over hours, days, and even weeks. It is beyond the remit of this text to go into this in more detail but as the example above illustrates, the common pitfalls are:

- Failure to gather adequate information.
- Failure to perform an adequate examination.
- Misinterpretation of findings at examination.
- Incorrect or incomplete investigations.
- Misinterpretation of investigation results—even experts may disagree on the findings on an apparently simple investigation such as a chest X-ray. In studies of the accuracy of radiological procedures amongst experienced

radiologists interobserver error ranged from 9 to 24% and intra-observer error from 3 to 31%. This was first studied by Garland in the 1950s and has been reconfirmed many times since.[11] Garland wrote 'In evaluating pairs of roentgenograms, one experienced physician is apt to disagree with another in about one third of the cases and (on review) to disagree with himself in one fifth of them.'

♦ Ignorance or inexperience, and in particular one's failure to recognize them.

♦ Inability to keep an open mind when patterns do not fit. If things don't feel right then they probably aren't and when all else fails, go back to the beginning and take a proper history and examination and reassess all of the information with an experienced colleague.

Why do we make diagnostic errors?

In addition to these pitfalls resulting from inadequate performance, attempts have been made to define the psychological factors that influence diagnostic decisions.[12] Most of us employ shortcuts (heuristics) when we assess patients—indeed it would be impossible to see 20 patients in a clinic without so doing. Using shortcuts is an acquired skill and depends on the ability to recognize patterns and significant deviations from normality. Some of the common errors that arise in diagnosis fall into the following categories.

Familiarity and playing the numbers game

All of us estimate the likelihood of a disease being present—probably without ever having formally read any relevant epidemiological studies. However, it is not unreasonable to assume that common things arise commonly. So, during an influenza epidemic a primary care physician seeing large numbers of patients with headache, fever, and muscle aches and pains may all too easily make a short-cut diagnosis of influenza rather than early meningococcal meningitis because he has seen eight similar cases in the last 48 hours and meningitis is so much rarer. The annual legal reports of the medical defence unions show that this is a recurring problem.

Jumping to conclusions too early on and sticking with that conclusion even in the face of conflicting information ('mind-lock')

It is a sobering experience to go back through the notes and review your own decision-making in cases that were either misdiagnosed or that took a long time to unravel. This author has found himself on a number of occasions wondering how he could ever have stuck with a particular line of thought for so long when with hindsight sufficient information was present at the outset.

Reaching a diagnosis too early may hinder the ability to change course even when the weight of evidence indicates you should. I believe it is much better to keep an open mind and say 'I don't know the diagnosis here' than to force thinking along lines that you and others may later have difficulty abandoning.

Over-reliance on specific information that leads to 'premature closure'

This is another pitfall similar to 'mind lock'. It is often seen with the interpretation of diagnostic tests—'it can't be a pulmonary embolism because the D-dimer is not elevated,' or 'the CT scan is normal so this isn't a subarachnoid haemorrhage'.

The framing effect

The way in which information is presented can also have a significant impact on the way in which it is interpreted. This is often seen in handovers and referrals. 'Please see this frequent attender with chronic fatigue, hyperventilation and vaso-vagal syncope'—a patient who in fact turned out to have Addison's disease and severe postural hypotension but several clinicians missed the point perhaps because of the pejorative way in which the referral was initially phrased.

Errors in drug prescribing and administration

Prescribing medication, along with surgical intervention, constitutes the largest source of error in medical practice. Every day in the UK some 2.5 million prescriptions are written, of which about 10% are subject to error of some sort. The majority of these result in no harm to patients either because systems are in place to pick them up (e.g. checking by nursing and pharmacy staff) or because they are of a relatively minor nature (e.g. omission of a drug or incorrect timing of administration). However, a number of studies from different countries have consistently shown that about 6.5% of all emergency admissions to hospital are as a direct result of adverse reactions to drugs and of these 9% are clearly preventable and 63% possibly preventable.[13,14] This adds up to about 250 000 admissions a year in the UK alone. Hospital inpatients fair little better, with about 10% suffering adverse drug reactions after admission, of which 1 in 8 are of sufficient severity to merit reporting to the UK MHRA yellow card reporting system.[15] To paraphrase Charlton Heston who as president of the National Rifle Association once famously said 'Guns don't kill people—*people* kill people', think of it as 'drugs don't kill people—*prescribers* kill people'.

The prescribing process can be broken down into a number of stages whereby error may occur at each stage.

The decision to prescribe

As discussed it is very hard to quantify the error rate in diagnosis that leads to inappropriate prescribing. Making a decision to prescribe demands a complex risk–benefit analysis that is dependent on accurate information on the following:

- the diagnosis
- an understanding of the natural history and severity of the condition if left untreated
- the patient's physiology and co-morbidity (e.g. renal failure, pregnancy)
- the patient's previous experience with medication, including drug allergies and intolerances
- the evidence for the effectiveness of the drug proposed
- the value of the benefit of the drug
- the incidence of side-effects of the drug
- the severity of the side-effects of the drug
- other drugs that the patient may be receiving and the likelihood for interactions to occur
- the applicability of clinical trials data to the patient in question
- the cost-effectiveness of the drug.

Clearly all of these steps are subject to error, lack of information, ignorance, and misinformation, which may have a serious impact on the decision to prescribe. In many areas of medicine one has to learn to make judgements in the absence of adequate information.

The multiple dimensions of risk assessment

Most prescribers struggle to weigh a common but relatively minor side-effect of a drug against a rare but devastating one. However, the balance is not a simple two-dimensional trade-off between frequency and severity of adverse effects—greater risks of adverse outcomes are taken when the underlying disease is itself more severe. Hence a remedy for a common cold should have no common side-effects and any severe side-effect must be vanishingly rare because the disease severity does not justify the risk involved, however small. Contrast that with the widespread use of cytotoxic chemotherapy for aggressive malignancy where the incidence of drug-induced nausea and vomiting may be 100% and bone marrow suppression and life-threatening infection are common. Untreated, the risk of death is almost certain and hence the balance tips in favour of treatment despite the attendant risks. The other dimension that comes into play is the efficacy of the treatment. A toxic drug regimen that achieves cure or prolonged remission is more likely to find acceptance than one that has only marginal benefits.

Having weighed up all of the available information, then a specific drug needs to be chosen with the most appropriate dosage, route of administration, and duration of treatment. Drug treatment must then be monitored to ensure the expected benefits are realized as well as to pick up side-effects and to titrate dosage.[16]

Few studies have addressed the quality of the risk assessment process that underpins prescribing as a source of adverse outcomes and most focus on the downstream problems that arise once the decision to write the prescription has been made. The 2007 NPSA[13] report—'Safety in doses: medication safety incidents in the NHS' is a good source of up-to-date information.

The drug history

A full drug history must be taken from every patient and collateral information sought if necessary. Details should include current drug treatment, including self-medication and use of non-prescription products such as herbal and traditional medicines. All patients should be asked about drug intolerance and allergy. The term hyper-susceptibility rather than allergy may be preferable as many significant drug reactions do not involve true allergic mechanisms, but 'allergy' is in common usage. If a patient reports intolerance to a drug then establish the nature of the event. All drug intolerance should be clearly recorded in the patient record and the patient's history of intolerance must be checked at every stage of the prescribing and administration process.

> All drug charts and medical records should be clearly marked to identify all known drug intolerance—if there are none known then the entries should state 'no known medicine intolerance'.[13]

The use of red alert wrist bracelets in hospital for patients with known drug allergies may help to heighten awareness and prompt further checking before drugs are administered—but they are not infallible.

> If you do not know the patient's drug history and it is not documented you must not prescribe, dispense, or administer a medicine.[13]

Antibiotics are widely used and allergies to them, especially penicillins are common. Even though an allergy to penicillin may be correctly documented on the drug chart, errors still occur with depressing frequency.

In 2001, in Bradford, a 38-year-old woman suffered an anaphylactic reaction, cardiac arrest, and subsequent brain damage from which she later died, when she was administered Magnapen® despite the fact that her notes stated she had a previous allergic reaction to penicillin and she was wearing a red allergy wrist band. The staff looking after her failed to realize that Magnapen® is the trade name for co-fluampicil and contains a combination of two penicillin-based drugs.

A similar misunderstanding occurs with the combination of piperacillin and tazobactam (Tazocin®). In a recent set of interviews for specialist training posts this author found that only four of 12 candidates presented with a real drug chart clearly stating penicillin allergy realized that Tazocin® was inappropriately prescribed.

Other drugs commonly implicated in a failure to heed previous episodes of intolerance are opioid analgesic agents and non-steroidal anti-inflammatory drugs.

The prescription

That doctors' handwriting is often illegible has long been the source of amusement but sadly poor writing, inappropriate abbreviations, and sloppy practice still results in significant error on a daily basis. Electronic prescribing (see below) eliminates problems due to illegibility but it is not yet universally available. There is no defence for poor handwriting that introduces doubt or error into the prescribing process.

Look-alike or sound-alike drug names

Particular care must be used when prescribing a drug that sounds or looks similar to another product when handwritten. Hydralazine and hydroxyzine, amiodarone and amlodipine, bisoprolol and bisacodyl have all been confused. Problems with look-alike drugs compounded with bad writing skills may be eliminated by electronic prescribing, but if you select the wrong drug name from a drop-down list because it sounds like the drug you want, then an electronic system is unlikely to be of help.

Inappropriate abbreviation or symbol

The Institute for Safe Medication Practices (http://www.ismp.org) has produced a list of error-prone abbreviations, symbols, and dose designations.

Perhaps the most commonly seen potential problems are with confusion between nanograms (e.g. calcitriol), micrograms (digoxin), and milligrams if the abbreviations ng, μg, and mg are used. Never abbreviate 'nano' or 'micro'; always write these out in full.

Poorly written prescriptions for insulin and heparin continue to threaten patient safety. A rushed entry for heparin 5000U can look very much like heparin 50000 with potentially catastrophic results. Never abbreviate 'units' to 'U'; write it out in full.

The prescription for insulatard shown in Fig. 2.6 is intended to be 20 units but the use of the abbreviation U for units combined with sloppy writing gives the impression that 200 units are required. Fortunately, as this was on a discharge prescription the pharmacist picked up the problem and rectified it before harm occurred.

Wrong formulation

The way in which a drug is formulated influences the kinetics of absorption and this is exploited by manufacturers in an attempt to achieve specific absorption profiles. Hence short-, intermediate-, and long-acting insulins have been developed to achieve glycaemic control in different settings. Unless the prescriber is aware of the different formulations available they will run the risk of exposing their patients to greater risks of poor glycaemic control.

A patient was inadvertently prescribed 20 units of Humulin S® (short-acting soluble insulin) instead of their usual Humulin I® (intermediate-acting isophane insulin) and as a result became profoundly hypoglycaemic.

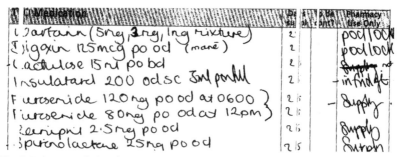

Fig. 2.6 The prescription for insulatard is intended to be 20 units but the use of the abbreviation U for units combined with sloppy writing (the 'u' looks like a '0') gives the impression that 200 units are required!

Wrong route of administration

Many drugs can be given by a variety of routes, but often the dosage appropriate for one route is inappropriate for another. In other cases drugs have been administered by a route that is never appropriate. This is a recurrent source of significant morbidity.

> In 2004, shortly after delivery, a 30-year-old woman died when she was given the local anaesthetic agent bupivacaine intravenously instead of via an epidural injection. The verdict of unlawful killing in 2008 was the first of its kind against an NHS Trust.

Dispensing

Fewer errors appear to occur in the dispensing process than in prescribing and administering medicines, perhaps because the culture of pharmacy is more safety aware and operating procedures are more stringently applied. The rates of error are about 0.1%, and most of these are picked up before the drug is dispensed to the patient.[13] However, serious problems can and do occur if the wrong medication or dosage is inadvertently supplied.

Preparation

Some medications require a degree of preparation before they are administered and this additional step is commonly subject to error. Preparation may involve calculations and dilutions and experience shows that this is a particularly hazardous process. Problems are even more likely to occur in paediatric practice because of dosage adjustments at different ages and weights.

Try the example below and imagine doing it in a clinical setting where a patient is rapidly deteriorating and time is of the essence. It is your first day in a new hospital as a junior doctor on ITU.

> A patient with severe septic shock requires an intravenous infusion of noradrenaline and you are asked to give a solution containing 80 micrograms of noradrenaline acid tartrate per ml at a rate of 0.2 ml per minute through a central venous line using a drip counter. You are given a vial containing 2 mg per ml noradrenaline acid tartrate and a bag containing 500 ml 5% dextrose. Calculate this without looking at the answer at the end of the chapter!

Never attempt to do this in reality without using manufacturer or departmental guidelines or referring to the British National Formulary (appendix 6 relating to intravenous additives) and asking someone to check your calculation independently. In addition to this, there are systems available whereby dilutions and infusion rates for commonly administered agents are pre-programmed into infusion devices thereby providing both a routine check on calculations but also a tool to audit accuracy and deviations from protocols.

Administration

Administration errors may arise for a variety of reasons but commonly from a simple lack of concentration and failure to have adequate checks in place.

Confusion between furosemide (prescribed 160 mg as 4 tablets of 40 mg) and gliclazide led to one patient receiving 320 mg gliclazide. The packaging is similar (Fig. 2.7) and it is easy to see how an error was made. The patient was symptomatically severely hypoglycaemic and required a total of 650 mg dextrose in 48 hours but made an uneventful recovery.

Pre-prepared infusions may reduce the potential for miscalculation in achieving the correct dilutions and also reduce the risk of contamination but problems may arise when packaging is not sufficiently distinctive and failures in storage and checking occur (Fig. 2.8). A nurse inadvertently picked up

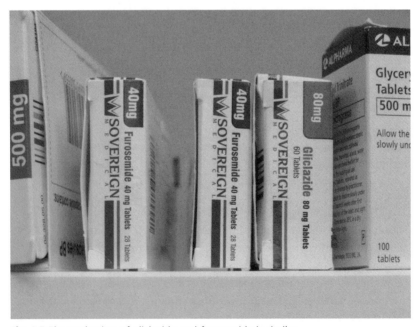

Fig. 2.7 The packaging of gliclazide and furosemide is similar.

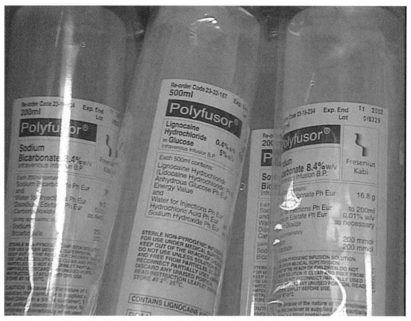

Fig. 2.8 A patient died when a nurse inadvertently picked up a pre-prepared infusion bag of lignocaine (lidocaine) instead of the sodium bicarbonate. The packaging is clearly not sufficiently distinctive to prevent this error from occurring again.

a pre-prepared infusion bag of lignocaine (lidocaine) instead of the sodium bicarbonate that had been prescribed, and as a result a patient had a cardiac arrest. The error was only detected at the time of the cardiac arrest when it was too late and the patient died.

> Never interrupt someone who is preparing or administering a drug—momentary disruption of concentration may lead to error. In some hospitals, nurses doing their drug rounds wear a bright tabard with a logo indicating they must not be disturbed, reinforcing the importance of their role to both their colleagues, their patients, and to themselves.

Patient information

Safe prescribing demands that the recipient understands and agrees to their role in the process and all prescribers need to be proficient in counselling patients or their carers about their drug treatment. It stands to reason that without such agreement and understanding adherence to treatment is likely to be low. Some drug regimens are complex and require a high level of co-operation from the patient and it is essential to provide clear information—ideally in the form of a patient information letter.

> An 80-year-old woman was receiving digoxin at a dose of 62.5 micrograms and her GP asked her to take two tablets a day until she received her new prescription and he amended the label on her tablet bottle. Two weeks later he wrote a prescription for digoxin 125 micrograms once a day but the patient put her new tablets into the old container and continued to take two tablets a day. She developed digoxin toxicity and had to be admitted to hospital as an emergency.

In some circumstances it may be necessary to advise that patients carry a warning card (e.g. a steroid card or anticoagulation booklet) or wear an alert bracelet or tag (e.g. warning of a serious adverse drug reaction such as anaphylaxis).

Monitoring

Over 80% of all drugs are prescribed on a repeat basis and it is an essential part of prescribing that monitoring is done carefully. Good monitoring ensures that drugs that are ineffective can be stopped, dosages can be titrated, adverse effects detected, adherence to treatment assessed, and the need for continuing treatment reviewed. Not surprisingly it can be a complex process and it is an area where shortcomings can have serious results.

> A 79-year-old woman was prescribed warfarin for atrial fibrillation. She developed back pain and visited her GP over a period of several weeks when blood tests were performed and a combination of paracetamol and non-steroidal anti-inflammatory drugs were prescribed. The patient assumed the pain killers were appropriate and that the blood tests included regular INR measurements but in fact the GP had forgotten she was receiving warfarin. When she developed extensive bruising the INR was finally measured and found to be greater than 10. The non-steroidal anti-inflammatory drugs were stopped and the dosage of warfarin reduced and regular monitoring was reinstated.

Reducing errors in blood transfusion

As we have already seen, accurate patient identification is crucial in avoiding error. Nowhere is this more relevant than in blood transfusion where incorrect transfusion remains a source of significant harm. Between 1996 and 2006 the UK Serious Hazards of Transfusion haemovigilance scheme (http://www.shot-uk.org) received 3763 reports, of which 2717 (72%) related to incorrect blood component transfusion (ICBT). Twenty-four patients died and 100 suffered major morbidity. The single biggest reason for these errors is incorrect patient identification.[17]

Why is it so hard to get this right? Although none of it is intellectually demanding it is a complex process and there are numerous stages at which checking is required and where errors may be introduced:

Error-prone stages in the blood transfusion process

- Ensuring the blood sample and result that trigger the decision to transfuse come from the correct patient
- Identifying the patient from whom the sample for cross-matching is taken
- Taking the blood and labelling it correctly
- Laboratory processing
- Taking cross-matched blood from storage refrigerators
- Checking patient identification before administering blood
- Monitoring patients during and after transfusion

Staff can become complacent with routine tasks, they may be distracted by other events, and they may be inadequately trained.

In response to this, end-to-end computerized control of transfusion has been very successfully introduced.[17,18] The system is designed around bar code patient identification to simplify and guide the user through every step of the process. All the patient identification is electronically controlled at every stage. When the laboratory has released the cross-matched blood, the patient wrist band is scanned and the computer prints off a sticker. The cross-matched blood cannot be taken from the refrigerator without the code from the sticker and only the correct blood can be delivered to the clinical area. The system allows accurate audit and can also incorporate a decision-support facility that may help reduce unnecessary transfusion requests. However, no system is failsafe—in operating theatres wrist bands are sometimes cut off to allow access to forearm veins for cannulation, and the barcode is separated from the patient. In the future, biometric identification with fingerprints or iris scans may be viable.

Intravenous drug administration

Ensuring safe intravenous administration of drugs also poses serious challenges particularly if some degree of preparation of the product is required before administration (e.g. dissolution and/or dilution). Administration of intravenous medicines is subject to error at least 25% more often than oral medicines and when mistakes occur they are more likely to cause death or serious harm.[13]

Let us return to the dosage calculation posed above with severe shock requiring an intravenous infusion of noradrenaline.

> A patient with severe septic shock requires an intravenous infusion of noradrenaline and you are asked to give a solution containing 80 micrograms of noradrenaline acid tartrate per ml at a rate of 0.2 ml per minute through a central venous line using a drip counter. You are given a vial containing 2 mg per ml noradrenaline acid tartrate and a bag containing 500 ml 5% dextrose.

> The answer is to add 40 mg of noradrenaline acid tartrate (20 ml of solution) to 480 ml of 5% dextrose to achieve a mixture containing 40 mg per 500 ml. This is 80 micrograms per ml. This is then run through a drip counter at 0.2 ml per min.

It is easy to see how you might make the wrong calculation in the heat of the moment, pick the wrong diluent, give it at the wrong rate or maybe be asked to set up an infusion using a pump (generously donated by the League of Friends) you have never seen before. How can this process be simplified and thereby made safer?

Equipment needs to be readily available and standardized so that the training and experience you received to use infusion pumps during your 4 months in medicine is relevant to your next 4 months in oncology. Far too often responsibility for equipment purchasing is devolved down to ward level resulting in a bewildering array of incompatible equipment even within a single hospital. Training then becomes fragmented. Never assume you can work out how to use equipment you have never seen before—the consequences of getting it wrong are not the same as getting the wrong ring tone on your new mobile phone.

Pumps need to be programmed and we all know how simple it is to make a basic error with keypad numbers. When did you last dial a wrong number? Tapping in the decimal point incorrectly for the infusion rate of noradrenaline might well kill someone. Smart pumps now exist that store pre-programmed infusion rates. Units can decide which pre-programmed information the pumps should store allowing them to build up a formulary of drugs and locally agreed appropriate concentrations and infusion rates. In this way a simple error with the keypad will not allow delivery of drug infusions that are outside acceptable tolerances.

Most units where intravenous drugs are regularly prepared and administered have guidelines and protocols for ensuring the correct drug, correct diluent, correct dosage, and correct infusion rate are utilized. Make sure you follow these and if you are not familiar with them then ask a more experienced colleague to assist you. Never place yourself or your patient in the situation of having to give a potentially toxic drug when you have never done it before and you have not received adequate training and supervision. Most departments that use standard dosages of intravenous infusions make use of pre-prepared infusion bags that come from a commercial producer or the pharmacy department. This significantly reduces the potential for dilutional errors, and minimizes contamination. It is particularly relevant for chemotherapeutic regimens.

Errors in the operating theatre

The operating theatre is a potentially hazardous environment. While each individual surgical specialty has its own unique set of potential errors that may lead to adverse events, many potential 'sites' of error and injury are shared across surgical specialties. Whether you are a neurosurgeon, a urologist, or a colorectal surgeon, patients can be harmed during the process of transferring them on and off the operating table and they may suffer harm while on the operating table in the form of developing pressure sores, nerve palsies, compartment syndrome, DVTs, and pulmonary emboli, and infective complications of surgery. Similarly, no surgical specialty is immune from wrong patient and wrong site surgery or of the problem of retained swabs and instruments. These latter topics and methods to prevent them are discussed in great detail in Chapter 7.

Patient transfer on and off the operating table

Errors can lead to harm during the process of positioning the patient on the operating table and during transfer of the patient off the operating table at the end of the operation.

First, the patient must be safely transferred from trolley to operating table. Patients have fallen off the trolley during this process because the brakes of either the trolley or the operating table had not been applied. Serious harm has occurred in such cases. A few years ago an elderly female patient was being transferred on to a radiology table for an X-ray to be done. No one checked to see if the brakes on the wheels of the trolley were on—they had not been applied. The patient fell, fracturing her hip. This was internally fixed. During the postoperative period she developed pneumonia and died.

Intravenous and arterial lines have been dislodged during the transfer process from trolley to table. These need to be carefully secured and protected during the transfer process. The same applies to endotracheal tubes, as the consequences of displacement may be disastrous.

Errors leading to adverse events occurring while on the operating table

Once on the operating table the patient can sustain harm from a number of sources:

- the skin is vulnerable to development of pressure sores
- diathermy burns can arise from contact with electrically grounded metal objects
- the lower limbs are at risk from compartment syndrome
- nerve palsies in the arms and legs may occur
- arms and particularly legs supported in leg stirrups, can collapse (limb fractures and other serious injuries have been reported)
- DVTs may develop while the patient is on the operating table, leading subsequently to a pulmonary embolus.

The use of diathermy

There are several do's and don'ts when it comes to the use of diathermy. An electrosurgical procedure safety checklist:

- *Do's*
  - avoid placing the grounding pad near scars or the sites of implants (hip prostheses, cardiac pacemakers)
  - place the ground plate as close to the operative site as possible and preferably over well vascularized muscular areas
  - shave, clean, and dry the site of the ground pad (excess hair is the commonest cause of electrosurgical burns)
  - check the ground plate is in good contact with the patient
  - recheck the plate contact and cable connection whenever the patient has been moved

- ensure the patient is not in contact with any metal (drip stands, metal components of the operating table, such as the leg stirrups)
- place the active electrode in a holder when not in use
- moisten swabs with saline.

◆ *Don'ts*

- use monopolar diathermy near structures with end-arteries, e.g. the penis (a high concentration of current in the base of the penis can cause injury to the artery)
- allow fluid to pool near the ground plate
- locate the ground plate over bony points, scars, implanted prostheses
- use bent or crumpled plates.

The skin can be burnt as a consequence of pools of flammable, alcohol-based skin preparation fluid catching fire when the diathermy is applied near the pools of fluid. This problem is best avoided by not using alcohol-based cleaning solutions.

Paraffin-based skin creams are flammable and, therefore, they also have the potential to ignite when a diathermy current is applied near them.

Dry swabs are also flammable and can catch fire from a diathermy spark.

A 4-year-old boy was injured in this way at Lancaster hospital. He had been admitted for maxillofacial surgery. The surgeon was using diathermy and he turned away from the patient for a moment to prepare the implant. While his attention was directed away from the patient a spark from the diathermy had started a fire on one of the dry swabs in the little boy's mouth. By the time the surgeon looked back there were flames coming out of the boy's mouth. He suffered severe injuries to the inside of his mouth and his lips.

Harm related to patient positioning

Lower limb compartment syndrome

This is a relatively rare problem, but the consequences of a missed diagnosis can be very serious—a limb may be permanently damaged and the mortality from delayed relief of a compartment syndrome is considerable. It is characterized by raised pressure within an unyielding osteofascial compartment, which if sustained reduces capillary perfusion below a level necessary for tissue viability, and as a consequence leads to irreversible muscle and nerve damage. Prompt decompression of the affected compartment(s) by fasciotomy is necessary in order to prevent irreversible ischaemic necrosis of the muscles and nerves of the compartment. It is classically caused by trauma to a limb, revascularization after a period of ischaemia, burns, or exercise, but it is also well described in the leg in association with the lithotomy position.

Any factor that induces ischaemia in the leg can lead to a compartment syndrome. Ischaemia disrupts the integrity of the vascular endothelium, leading to fluid shifts into the extracellular tissue space with a consequent rise in tissue pressure. Lower limb compartment syndrome occurs with a frequency in the order of 1 in 3500 in association with the lithotomy position.[19]

Presentation and treatment

The classic presentation is with pain (typically out of all proportion to the injury and to the physical signs) and paraesthesia in the leg. Passive stretching of the affected muscles exacerbates the pain. Even an epidural anaesthetic and large doses of intravenous opiates may fail to control the pain. Sensory loss in the distribution of the nerves traversing the affected compartments may be a useful early sign. The skin may be pink and peripheral pulses may well still be present. It is possible to measure compartment pressures, but the equipment for doing this and expertise in recording and interpreting the pressures so measured are not always readily available. A high index of suspicion is therefore required to make a clinical diagnosis.

Prevention

So, try to avoid the conditions that predispose to compartment syndrome.[20] If using the lithotomy position, use a low lithotomy as opposed to a high or exaggerated one. Try to avoid the Trendelenberg position (head down), again because this reduces perfusion pressure to the limb. Allen stirrups are said to cause less elevation of calf pressure than calf supports. Avoid dorsiflexion of the ankle (this elevates calf compartment pressure). Ensure that the anaesthetist maintains normovolaemia and blood pressure. The major factor determining the likelihood of development of a lower limb compartment syndrome is time spent in the lithotomy position. For long procedures (>4 hours) consider lowering the legs from the elevated position for a short while, to enhance tissue perfusion.

Pressure or traction induced nerve palsies

A number of nerves are at risk of damage during the course of an operation, as a consequence of pressure effects from retractors or because of the position of the limbs or pressure from the operating table, e.g. femoral neuropathy due to inappropriate application of self-retaining retractors.

The ulnar nerve can sustain a traction injury leading to an ulnar nerve palsy if positioned at more than a 90-degree angle from the chest.[21] One of the authors performed a cystectomy on a patient. The procedure lasted 4 hours.

The patient's arm was maintained in a 90-degree abducted position for the duration of the operation. After the operation, despite having had his bladder removed through a long midline incision, his main concern was severe pain and pins and needles in the distribution of the ulnar nerve. The pins and needles persisted for 12 months!

A host of intra-abdominal and retroperitoneal nerves may be injured by pressure from the blades of retractors. A pressure injury to the femoral nerve can be prevented by following the advice of Burnett and Brendler[22] who state that:

> after positioning of a self-retaining retractor, the surgeon should insert the fingers beneath the retractor blades bilaterally to be sure that there is clearance between the ends of the retractor and the psoas muscle. The spermatic cords should not be retracted and should be visualized below the lateral edges of the retractor, further ensuring that the psoas muscles and underlying femoral nerves are not being compressed.

Other nerves at risk from compression by retractor blades include the lateral femoral cutaneous nerve of the thigh, the ilioinguinal nerve, and the genitofemoral nerve.

Pressure point protection

Certain points of the body are at risk of necrosis from prolonged pressure contact with operating tables—the back of the head, the scapula, the sacrum, and the heels. Place 'gel' pads at all these pressure points (Fig. 2.9).

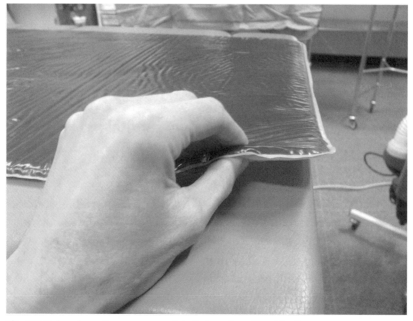

Fig. 2.9 Gel pads under pressure points help reduce the risk of pressure sores.

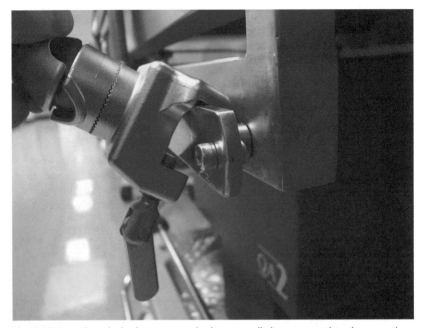

Fig. 2.10 Even though the leg supports had supposedly been secured to the operating table, when the surgeon checked it proved possible, with minimal force, to detach the leg support.These particular leg supports had not been specifically designed for the particular type of operating table - but there was nothing to prevent their use on the wrong table! **Always check yourself that the leg is secure**.

Leg supports that give way

The leg supports that hold the legs in position can give way if not adequately tightened or secured to the operating table. Check that the supports are secure and that they will hold your own weight (Fig. 2.10).

Generic safety checks prior to any surgical procedure

- ◆ Ensure the correct patient identification and the correct side and site of the operation.
- ◆ Safely transfer the patient on and off the operating table—brakes on, adequate staff, transfer 'downhill' rather than 'uphill', and avoid inadvertent tube and line removal.
- ◆ Position the patient safely on the table—avoid metal contact, pad pressure points with 'gel' pads (Fig. 2.9), position the lower limbs as flat as possible to avoid lower limb compartment syndrome.

- Skin preparation—avoid alcohol-based fluids, especially in the region of mucous membranes, eg. genital region; avoid pooling of inflammable liquids, if used.
- Give DVT and antibiotic prophylaxis.

Failure to give DVT prophylaxis

DVTs and pulmonary emboli are the commonest, most major potentially avoidable postoperative problem in surgical patients and every surgeon must take appropriate precautions to prevent their occurrence. A recent House of Commons Select Committee[8] has reported that a substantial number of hospitalized patients, many of them undergoing surgery, do not receive measures to prevent DVTs and pulmonary emboli and then subsequently develop a DVT or pulmonary emboli. We know from our own audit of 100 surgical procedures that in one-third of patients the surgeon and anaesthetist did not administer appropriate DVT prophylaxis at the time of operation—either through lack of knowledge of our own guidelines or simply because they forgot to do so.

In the UK, the National Institute for Clinical Excellence (NICE) has recently issued guidelines on DVT prophylaxis and in the USA the American College of Chest Physicians publishes very comprehensive evidence-based guidelines review of all aspects of thromboembolic disease prevention and treatment: *Guidelines on Antithrombotic and Thrombolytic Treatment.*[23] Using either set of guidelines appropriately would go some considerable way to ensuring that deaths and morbidity from VTE could be reduced.

The American College of Chest Physicians guidelines categorize patients into three groups according to their risk of VTE (see Table 2.1) and make recommendations on the required degree of DVT prophylaxis. It is important to remember that 'minor surgery' is defined by these guidelines as any procedure taking less than 30 minutes and major surgery as any procedure taking more than 30 minutes. Many patients undergoing operations such as circumcision or hernia repair (what many surgeons would regard as pretty minor surgery) will be on the operating table for longer that 30 minutes, so instantly these patients are elevated from a low-risk category of minor surgery, into a moderate risk category. DVT prevention should be adjusted accordingly.

Failure to give antibiotic prophylaxis

A comprehensive review of antibiotic prophylaxis for the prevention of postoperative infections is beyond the scope of this book. However, it is important to emphasize that no antibiotic prophylaxis policy is of any value whatsoever if the operating surgeon fails to double check that the anaesthetist has given the antibiotic prophylaxis. Again, from our own audit of 100 surgical procedures, in 1 in 10 patients the surgeon and anaesthetist forgot to administer appropriate antibiotic prophylaxis (appropriate as determined by our own guidelines) at the time of operation, again either through lack of knowledge of the guidelines or simply because they forgot to do so. A gentle reminder from the observer ensured the antibiotics were given.

Our experience of failure to give antibiotic prophylaxis prior to surgical operations is not unique. Bratzler *et al.*[24] reported that only 56% of patients had antibiotic prophylaxis within 1 hour of the start of the operation. Only 41% discontinued within 24 hours, thereby increasing the risk of antibiotic-resistant organisms and *C. difficile* infection.

Errors in the postoperative period

Failure to ask advice where appropriate and inappropriate delegation

The days of junior doctors operating unsupervised are numbered because of their relative inexperience. Increasingly, the consultant is in attendance for emergency procedures as well as for elective ones. However, some consultant surgeons continue to delegate operations to junior surgeons who are not capable of performing such procedures safely, and who unfortunately do not have the insight to appreciate this. As a consultant, if you delegate operations to junior surgeons—elective or emergency—do make sure that the operation is within the capabilities of that junior surgeon and make sure that the surgeon knows you are very happy to come in and assist at a moments notice. If you are not in a position to be immediately available, ensure that a named consultant colleague is and that the operating junior surgeon, anaesthetist, and theatre staff know who that consultant is. As a junior surgeon, make sure you know who is covering you and how to get hold of them should a problem develop during the operation for which you need help.

Day to day care

It is the consultant's responsibility to make sure that the junior staff have adequate skills and expertise. A proper scheme of supervision within the surgical team is essential so that general management and a knowledge of symptoms and signs of complications can be taught. Make sure that inappropriate delegation does not occur, where an insufficiently experienced or knowledgeable doctor is expected to make decisions beyond his or her capability. A close system of communication must be set up and the junior staff must know that they are able to get in touch with their seniors at all times without fear of rebuff.

Make sure that your junior staff do at least a daily ward round and write daily follow-up notes during the postoperative period, recording any significant events. Be particularly wary at weekends when fewer senior doctors are available. Leaving junior doctors, particularly the inexperienced senior house officer, to care for a ward of patients for an entire weekend without some senior input can lead to problems. We can draw lessons from one particularly sad case— now known as the 'Southampton case'—which involved a young man who had undergone surgery to a fractured patella.[25] Over the course of the weekend following his operation, the patient developed sepsis. He was 'cared' for by two senior house officers working on a shift system. Neither doctor recognized the signs of septicaemia. They never suspected a possible infective cause for the patient's deterioration. At no stage was the patient reviewed by a senior doctor. The patient died of toxic shock syndrome. The two senior house officers were convicted of manslaughter on the basis that their care had amounted to gross negligence. Regular ward rounds by consultants, particularly at weekends, provides a safeguard against such catastrophes.

Shared care

Nowadays the care of individual patients is often shared between consultants. The surgeon who saw the patient in the clinic and booked the admission may therefore not be the consultant who actually carries out the operation. This is a situation that increases the risk of error, often because of simple communication issues. It therefore requires especial care to make sure that the patient gets the treatment he or she expected and has had explained. The process of consent needs particular attention.

One of the problems with shared care is the potential for the lack of a lead clinician whose responsibility it is to co-ordinate the patient's care. The fragmentation of care between specialists and subspecialists—often on hospital sites in different locations—is a particular problem here. Such a system runs the danger that no one single clinician has 'ownership' over the patient's care. There is no easy solution to this problem. One cause of this problem may be the move towards consultant surgeons being viewed as technicians rather than professionals.[26]

Medical devices

There are a plethora of medical and surgical devices that are used in day-to-day practice in hospitals and primary care where poor design can lead to error. It is not our intention to discuss the design faults of every possible device. Instead we will give the reader a flavour for some problems that are inherent to the design of devices that they may come across in practice.

Poorly designed equipment (hardware) can be a cause of error and accidents in all safety critical industries. The Three Mile Island nuclear power plant emergency was largely initiated and exacerbated by poor labelling of instrument panels, illogical design of those instrument panels, and inadequate data displays.

High reliability organizations nowadays have well developed equipment design standards, usability testing, and incident reporting systems to prevent and remedy design-induced errors. Unfortunately, while healthcare equipment is nowadays well designed and well tested for its usability, a poor culture of incident reporting has the potential to lead to delays in resolving problems.

We know that design-induced errors in the use of medical devices have led to patient injuries and deaths. User interfaces that are poorly designed can induce errors by even the most skilled users. So experts BEWARE!

The design of the user interface

Three case studies described below show how shortcomings in the design of the user interface can harm patients. As with so many potential sources of error in the healthcare setting, the capacity for the individual healthcare worker to change the system is inevitably limited (the authors are not immune to suffering from 'learned helplessness'!!), although this should not be taken to mean that the individual cannot make or initiate change. Our intention in describing these design errors in medical devices is to demonstrate to the individual reader the potential pitfalls that lie ahead. Armed with this knowledge, the individual can compensate for unsafe equipment, though clearly the long-term goal of any organization must be to purchase equipment that is designed with safety in mind.

Examples of design-induced errors

Oxygen flow control knob A physician was treating a patient with oxygen and set the flow control knob, as shown below to give 1.5 litres per minute. It was not clear to him that the machine would only give 1 or 2 litres per minute and there was no oxygen flow between the 1 and 2 setting. The knob rotated smoothly, suggesting that an intermediate setting was possible. The knob looked very similar in appearance to the controls of domestic cookers that do have intermediate settings.

The physician presumed, not unreasonably, that the control worked in the same way. The patient, an infant, became hypoxic before the error was discovered.

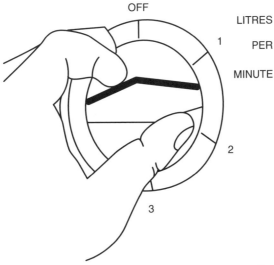

Fig. 2.11 Flow control knob for oxygen delivery. There is no oxygen flow between the 1 and 2 setting, but the smooth rotation of the knob between setting 1 and 2 gives the false impression that intermediate flows between 1 and 2 can be administered.

If the use of discrete rather than a continuous range of selectable values is inevitable given the nature of the equipment then a rotary control should be designed that clicks into the notched settings.

In this case the absence of data display giving the actual flow of oxygen being delivered was a critical failure.

Flow rate display An infusion device was fitted with a data display that was recessed into the face of the machine. When viewed from directly in front of the machine, the display could be read correctly. However, when viewed from the left-hand side, the first digit was concealed. The nurse thought that the patient was receiving 55 millilitres per minute. In fact 355 millilitres was being infused.

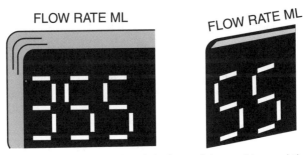

Fig. 2.12 View of the display from directly in front of the machine, and the view from an angle 40 degrees to the left.

Anaesthetic machine gave nitrous oxide instead of oxygen On 18 January 2001 a 3-year-old girl was rushed to a London hospital after suffering a fit at home. She had started fitting after receiving a flu jab at her GP practice.

Dr A, an A&E consultant, placed a mask on her face and turned a knob on the front of the anaesthetic machine to commence the flow of oxygen. However, instead of turning a white knob to release oxygen, he turned a blue knob, which released nitrous oxide. The machine did not have a display indicating whether it was administering oxygen or nitrous oxide.

A stressful crisis occurred during which the doctor did not consider the possibility that the girl was receiving nitrous oxide. As we shall see later in the book stressful crises often seem to induce 'perceptual narrowing', which impairs the operator's ability to consider alternative explanations for the problem they are encountering. After about 8 minutes the error was detected but by then the child had sustained severe hypoxic brain damage and she died later that evening.

In the past some orthopaedic procedures, such as reduction of fractures, were carried out in A&E departments using nitrous oxide, among other agents, as analgesia. The A&E department at the hospital was designed at a time in the early 1980s when piped nitrous oxide was recommended by NHS design standards. Those orthopaedic procedures are now carried out elsewhere and A&E units designed since the 1980s only have piped oxygen. The report into the death of the girl does not describe any risk management assessments about the presence of nitrous oxide in the department. Nor was there any mention of any induction training that the doctor had been given to warn him of the presence of nitrous oxide in such close proximity to oxygen.

User interface design: guidelines

A medical device that does not comply with the following guidelines may create hazards. If you believe that the design faults in any machine are hazardous you should make a report through the critical incident reporting systems.

1 The design should be consistent with user expectations, based on the user's previous experience with medical devices as well as established conventions about other hardware, such as domestic electrical equipment. Colour and shape coding, where appropriate, facilitates rapid identification of controls and displays.

2 Workstation, control, and display design should be compatible with the basic physical and intellectual capabilities of the user, such as strength,

dexterity, memory, reach, vision, and hearing. Auditory and visual signals should be loud and bright enough to be perceived by users working under various conditions of ambient noise and illumination.

3 Well laid out and uncluttered arrangements of controls and displays are essential. The association between a control and the relevant data display must be obvious. This facilitates proper identification and reduces the user's memory load. Ensure that the abbreviations, symbols, text, and acronyms placed on, or displayed by, the device are consistent with accepted standards.

4 With safety-critical mode selections, an independent status display must confirm what the machine is actually doing. It is not safe to rely on the operator looking at the selected switch or knob position to determine the mode in which the machine is operating.

5 Labels and displays should be easily read from typical viewing angles and distances. Symbol size, contrast, colour, and display depth are important considerations.

6 Knobs, switches, and keys should be designed and arranged in a way that reduces the likelihood of inadvertent activation, e.g. by brushing a switch and inadvertently turning it on. Make sure that controls provide tactile feedback.

Component installation

One of the most common problems reported in connection with medical devices is the improper connection of components and accessories. Some commonly reported errors are:

- tubing connected to the wrong port
- loose connections or accidental disconnections
- electrical leads inserted into an improper power source
- batteries or bulbs inserted incorrectly
- valves or other hardware installed backward or upside-down.

Injuries, deaths, and 'near misses' with ventilators have occurred because of disconnections of the breathing tubes due to poor tube and connector design. The situation is exacerbated because many manufacturers sell a wide range of accessories for a given type of device. There are a great variety of cables, leads, connectors, valves, and tubing on the market. Accessories for different models are often similar in appearance and/or difficult to install, leading to mis-installations and disconnections.

Guidelines

1 Cables, tubing, connectors, levers, and other hardware should be designed for easy installation and connection. If properly designed, incorrect installations should be impossible, extremely difficult, or so obvious that they can be easily detected and remedied.

2 User instructions should be understandable, and warnings conspicuous.

3 If a hazard cannot be eliminated by a design solution, colour codes or other markings will help the user achieve proper connections and component or accessory installation.

4 Positive locking mechanisms are desirable whenever the integrity of connections may be compromised by such factors as component durability, motion, or casual contact.

5 Protected electrical contacts (e.g. the conductors are recessed) are necessary for body leads that can be inadvertently introduced into outlets, power cords, extension cords, or other common connectors. If possible, exposed contacts should be avoided.

6 Components and accessories should be code numbered, so that defective ones can be replaced with the proper items.

Usability testing

A programme of usability testing should be set up to ensure that the average user can safely and effectively operate the device. The test should be carried out by the personnel who are going to be using the device and should be carried out under normal operational conditions.

This usability testing often reveals that the operators often actually use the device in a way that the designer had not envisaged. This can have major consequences. An example of this is illustrated in the following case study.

Case study: the Therac-25 high-energy radiotherapy machine

If you observe people who are using a piece of electronic equipment you will often see them select one particular operational mode of the equipment and then immediately realize that they should have selected another mode. They will then reselect the correct mode. This is a very common behaviour. We have all pressed fast-forward on a DVD/video player and then immediately pressed fast-rewind. This behaviour seems to be much more likely when one mode of the equipment is used more frequently than another.

The engineer who designed the Therac-25 radiotherapy machine had carried out all of the 1200 hours of testing of the machine himself. The machine had performed flawlessly during the testing.

It did not occur to the designer to observe ordinary operators operating the machine under normal operating conditions. Nor did he consider the consequences of a rapid reselection of mode. If such a test were carried out, it would have revealed a fatal design flaw in the Therac-25.

There were two modes in which the Therac-25 could function. The first was the low-energy mode in which an electron beam of about 200 rads was aimed at the patient and sent off in a short burst. The second mode was an X-ray mode, which used the full 25 million electron volt capacity of the machine. When the machine was switched into this second mode, a thick metal plate would move automatically between the beam source and the patient. As the electron beam passed through the plate, it was transformed into an X-ray beam that would then irradiate the tumours.

The problem was that when a mode reselection was made in less than 8 seconds, the software commanded the metal plate to withdraw, but the switch to a lower power did not occur. Although the machine told the operator it was in electron beam mode, it was actually in X-ray mode.

In 1986, Ray Cox, a Texas oil worker, went in for his usual radiation treatment for a tumour he had removed from his left shoulder. He had had this treatment eight times before. The technician got him set up on the table and went down the hall to start the treatment. Unfortunately, the technician made the fatal mode reselection error. As a result the patient received 125 times the desired amount of radiation.

In the treatment room, Ray was feeling repeated burning, stabbing pains on his back. None of the previous treatments had been like this. He cried out several times, asking whether the system was configured correctly but no one came to check on him. Finally, after the third painful burst, he got off the table, and went to the nurse's station.

Ray's health deteriorated rapidly from radiation burns and other complications from the treatment overdose. He kept in good humour about his condition, joking that 'Captain Kirk forgot to put his machine on stun'. He died 4 months later.

It is worth noting that the problem was not actually diagnosed until 3 weeks later, when it happened again to another patient. At this point, the senior technician realized something about the sequence of steps being taken must have been triggering the event. After investigation, he found the problem with the plate, and reported it to the manufacturer. Subsequent investigations showed that two other patients had died and three others were harmed as a result of this problem.

A further malevolent coincidence had contributed to this accident. There were two independent systems of communication between the treatment room and the control room, a video system and an audio intercom system. On the day of Ray's treatment both systems had failed. Had either of the systems been working, the patient's cries would probably have prompted the technician to stop the treatment earlier as it did in two of the other cases.

References

1 Wilson T, Sheikh A. Enhancing public safety in primary care. *Br Med J* 2002; **324**: 584–7.
2 Makeham MAB, Stromer S, Bridges-Webb C, *et al.* Patient safety events reported in general practice: a taxonomy. *Qual Saf Health Care* 2008; **17**: 53–7.
3 General Medical Council publications. *Good Medical Practice 2001.* www.gmc-uk.org/guidance/archive/gmp_2001.pdf/.
4 Royal College of Surgeons of England. *Good surgical practice.* Record keeping, p. 14. London; 2008. http://www.rcseng.ac.uk/rcseng/content/publications/docs/good-surgical-practice-1/.
5 Department of Health. *The Health Act 2006: Code of Practice for Prevention and Control of Healthcare Associated Infections.* London: Department of Health; 2006. http://www.dh.gov.uk/publications/.
6 Department of Health. *Saving lives: reducing infection, delivering clean and safe care document.* Department of Health; 2007. http://clean-safe-care.nhs.uk/.
7 National Audit Office. *The management and control of hospital acquired infection in acute NHS Trusts in England.* London: National Audit Office; 2000. http://www.nao.gov.uk/.
8 *The prevention of venous thromboembolism in hospitalised patients.* House of Commons Select Committee 23 February 2005. London: The Stationery Office Limited; 2005. http://www.parliament.uk/.
9 Fitzmaurice DA, Murray E. Thromboprophylaxis for adults in hospital. *Br Med J* 2007; **334**: 1017–18.
10 Brennan JM, Blair JE, Goonewardena S, *et al.* A comparison by medicine residents of physical examination versus hand-held ultrasound for estimation of right atrial pressure. *Am J Cardiol* 2007; **99**: 1614–16.
11 Garland LH. Studies on the accuracy of diagnostic procedures. *Am J Roentgenol* 1959; **82**: 25–38.
12 Redelmeier DA. The cognitive psychology of missed diagnoses. *Ann Intern Med* 2005; **142**: 115–20.
13 National Patient Safety Agency (NPSA). *Safety in doses: medication safety incidents in the NHS.* London: NPSA; 2007.
14 Pirmohamed M, James S, Meakin S, *et al.* Adverse drug reactions as cause of admission to hospital: prospective analysis of 18,820 patients. *Br Med J* 2004; **329**: 15–19.
15 Smith CC, Bennett PM, Pearce HM, *et al.* Adverse drug reactions in a hospital general medical unit meriting notification to the Committee on Safety of Medicines. *Br J Clin Pharmacol* 1996; **42**: 423–9.
16 Reynolds DJM. Practical prescribing. In: *Clinical pharmacology* (ed. DJM Reynolds) *Medicine,* Vol 36, p 360–363. Oxford: The Medicine Publishing Oxford 2003.

17 Davies A, Staves J, Kay J, Casbard A, Murphy MF. End to end electronic control of the hospital transfusion process to increase the safety of blood transfusions: strengths and weaknesses. *Transfusion* 2006; **46**: 352–64.

18 Staves J, Davies A, Kay J, *et al.* Electronic remote blood issue: a combination of remote blood issue with a system for end-to-end electronic control of transfusion to provide a 'total solution' for a safe and timely hospital blood transfusion service. *Transfusion* 2008; **48**: 415–24.

19 Halliwell JR, Hewitt BS, Joyner MH, Warner MA. Effect of various lithotomy positions on lower extremity pressure. *Anesthesiology* 1998; **89**: 1373–6.

20 Raza A, Byrne D, Townell N. Lower limb (Well leg) compartment syndrome after urological pelvic surgery. *J Urol* 2004; **171**: 5–11.

21 Cheney F. The American Society of Anesthesiologists Closed Claims Project: what we have learned, how it has affected practice, and how it will affect practice in the future. *Anesthesiology* 1999; **91**: 552–6.

22 Burnett AL, Brendler CB. Femoral neuropathy following major pelvic surgery: etiology and prevention. *J Urol* 1994; **151**: 163–5.

23 Proceedings of the Seventh ACCP Conference on Antithrombotic and Thrombolytic Therapy: evidence-based guidelines. *Chest* 2004; **126** (3 Suppl.): 172S–696S. http://www.nice.org.uk/guidance/index.jsp?action=byID&o=11006/.

24 Bratzler DW, Houck PM, Richards C, *et al.* Use of antimicrobial prophylaxis for major surgery: baseline results from the National Surgical Infection Prevention Project. *Arch Surg* 2005; **140**: 174–82.

25 Dyer C. Doctors face trial for manslaughter as criminal charges against doctors continue to rise. *Br Med J* 2002; **325**: 63.

26 Gannon C. Will the lead clinician please stand up? Personal view. *Br Med J* 2005; **330**: 737.

Further reading

Dovey SM, Meyers DS, Phillips RL Jr, *et al.* A preliminary taxonomy of medical errors in family practice. *Qual Saf Health Care* 2002; **11**: 233–8.

Pearse MF, Harry L, Nanchahal J. Acute compartment syndrome of the leg. *Br Med J* 2002; **325**: 557–8.

Report by the British Orthopaedic Association/British Association of Plastic Surgeons Working Party on the management of open tibial fractures. September 1997. *Br J Plast Surg* 1997; **50**: 570–83.

Add 40 mg of noradrenaline acid tartrate (20 ml of solution) to 480 ml of 5% dextrose to achieve a mixture containing 40 mg per 500 ml. This is 80 micrograms per ml. This is then run through a drip counter at 0.2 ml per min.

Chapter 3

Safety culture in high reliability organizations

In recent years, articles have appeared in medical journals drawing attention to the high rate of adverse events in healthcare and pointing out that healthcare seems to lack the safety systems and culture that exist in other safety-critical industries. A term that appears in many of these articles is high reliability organizations (HROs). Healthcare is compared unfavourably with HROs.

In an ideal world healthcare would find its own solutions to prevent clinical error. Indigenously developed healthcare safety systems would presumably have the advantage of having been designed from the start to allow for the many inherent complexities and uncertainties in the setting of healthcare.

However, we have been frustrated by the slow pace of change in the development of safety systems in healthcare. One solution would be to adopt and then adapt proven concepts from domains outside healthcare—namely the safety procedures used by HROs.

Many progressive healthcare organizations, particularly in the USA where litigation and compensation costs for preventable adverse events are high, have already started to use procedures developed from the techniques employed by HROs to enhance safety.

> It is very likely that in the next few years doctors will encounter an increasing number of patient safety initiatives that are based on HRO concepts. These doctors will probably have their own ideas about how relevant and appropriate to healthcare such concepts are. They will almost certainly hear their colleagues expressing views on the subject.
>
> A working knowledge of HRO concepts and working practices is therefore likely to be of benefit to all healthcare workers in the future.

High reliability organizations: background

In the 1970s and 1980s the attention of a number of organizational sociologists in various universities was drawn to the accident rates in certain organizations in a number of different industries. These accident rate statistics showed a consistent downward trend.

Since the 1990s some of these organizations have progressed further and have even managed to achieve a zero rate for major accidents over many consecutive years. For example, as of November 2008, UK-based airlines have not suffered an accident that has killed a passenger on board a British jet airliner for the best part of 20 years. Other first world countries have similar safety records. Thus, while accidents still happen in HROs, their ability to prevent catastrophic failure—indeed to turn it into success—is impressive.

Clearly, this safety success was not achieved because such organizations operate in an environment that is free from risk. Each HRO had suffered major catastrophes in the past and their operational environment had not suddenly become benign. In some cases, various developments in their operational environments have actually increased the risk of accidents. In the case of the commercial airline companies, for example, the airspace over major airports is busier than ever before, aviation authorities have authorized airliners to take off and land in very thick fog and the turn around time for the budget airlines is faster than ever before—and yet major accidents are extremely rare.

In other cases the organizations have decided (while in search of additional profit) to expose themselves to greater risk. For example, they have extended their activities into situations where more extreme or unpredictable weather occurred. The petroleum industry, for example, has been forced to search for oil in ever more hazardous environments such as beneath the Arctic Ocean.

One possible explanation for these safety improvements might have been that these organizations were merely using more reliable equipment. However, preliminary studies suggested that the improvements in safety performance exceeded the level that would have been achieved by improving the hardware alone. It seems as though these organizations have succeeded in making their employees more 'reliable': they have managed to prevent catastrophic *human errors*.

A conference at the University of Texas in April 1987 brought researchers together to focus attention on how HROs had managed to achieve their success. This conference had added poignancy because it took place exactly 1 year after the Chernobyl nuclear power station disaster and almost exactly 10 years after the terrible Tenerife air disaster.

Several important questions can be considered:

- Were these solutions *specific* to the industries that had developed them (and thus incapable of transfer to other domains)?
- If the solutions were not specific to the industries, to what extent could HRO concepts be transferred to other domains?
- Was there such a thing as a generic HRO that could be used as a starting point for transfer to other domains such as healthcare?

Initial research work into HROs was carried out at the University of California at Berkeley, the University of Michigan and George Washington University. At Berkeley, detailed research was carried out in air traffic control centres, a commercial nuclear power plant, and US Navy aircraft carriers.

Since the conference other organizations have been described as HROs as they also operate in high-risk environments and yet have demonstrated sustained improvements in their accident rates. They also seem to share similar features in their safety cultures. These organizations include commercial airlines, European and Japanese passenger railways, petroleum and chemical processing, and fire-fighting crews.

A case study in safety: US Navy Aircraft carrier—flight deck operations

During US Navy operational deployments, there are often up to 40 aircraft on the deck of a 'Nimitz' class aircraft carrier at any one time. Present on deck are up to 120 tons of high explosive ordnance and 120 tons of aviation fuel. Because of lack of space, aircraft have to be parked within 2 metres of each other, increasing the risk of any fire spreading rapidly. At any one time approximately 450 men will be loading bombs and missiles, refuelling, carrying out maintenance, and co-ordinating landings and take-offs.

In this fast moving and extremely noisy environment (so noisy that verbal communication is often impossible), deck personnel have to avoid being sucked into jet engine air intakes or being blown overboard by jet blast. They must also avoid the wires of the high-speed jet catapults that accelerate the jets at take off and the 'arrestor' cables that slow them down rapidly on landing. A man could be cut in half by these wires. There are over 60 000 take-offs and landings per year, night and day, in all weathers, within an extremely confined area. The 'icing on the cake' that makes this one of the most dangerous environments in any HRO is the fact that a few decks below this potentially explosive work site are the two nuclear reactors that power the vessel.

The flight deck of Nimitz class US Navy Aircraft carriers can therefore be seen as the archetypal 'high-risk' environment. One might imagine that accidents would occur frequently and would be catastrophic when they do occur.

In fact adverse incidents are rare and catastrophic events are extremely rare. Over the last 50 years there has been a continuous improvement in safety. In 1999 the number of class 'A' accidents (accidents with resulting costs in excess of $1 million) was 1.43 per 100 000 flight-hours compared with a rate of 55 in 1952. This is a reduction of more than 97%.

How has this been achieved? In brief (see below for detailed discussion) by:

- the use of standard operating procedures
- investigating accidents and near misses and instituting training to avoid these in future
- a culture of confidence and trust
- regular staff training in (a) technical skills, and (b) the role of human factors in error
- the use of *simple* safety systems ('nuts and bolts')
- personnel and process auditing
- open management and a balanced hierarchy where appropriate
- redundancy in hardware, personnel, and procedures.

Despite the fact that crew turnover is very high (virtually the entire deck crew will 'turnover' within 18 months), the US Navy is able to train all its staff in a very short time frame in these safety concepts and techniques. Very few of the crew have even a college level of education and so the US Navy does not have the luxury of being able to train university-educated personnel.

Thus, paradoxically this high-risk environment is virtually accident-free.

High reliability organizations: common features

Detailed studies[1-5] of HROs have identified some common general features. These features include:

- **A safety culture** in which individuals feel comfortable drawing attention to potential hazards or actual failures without fear of censure from management. There is a total determination to achieve consistently safe operations.

- **Analysis of operations.** There are regular audits to establish exactly what is going on at the 'frontline' and a very close attentiveness to the issues facing operators. HROs have reliable systems to monitor the level of compliance with required operating procedures.

- **Preoccupation with failure.** There is an acknowledgement of the high-risk, error-prone nature of an organization's activities and the expectation of failure at any time. The causes of errors and accidents are carefully analysed. HROs develop the capacity to detect unexpected threats and contain them before they cause harm.

- **Commitment to resilience.** HROs have regular exercises to practice recovery from serious accidents. These exercises help to dispel complacency in the work force that might otherwise result from having a very low rate of accidents.

In 1993 the UK's Health and Safety Commission gave a useful definition of a safety culture:

> The Safety Culture of an organisation is the product of the individual and group values, attitudes, competencies and patterns of behaviour that determine the commitment to and the style and proficiency of an organisation's health and safety programmes. Organisations with a positive safety culture are characterised by communications founded on mutual trust, by shared perceptions of the importance of safety and by confidence in the efficacy of preventive measures.

The consequences of failure

The organizations that developed into HROs had all suffered very costly accidents in the past. These costs included lives lost, physical losses to property, damaged reputations, and environmental damage. Examples include:

- The leak of toxic chemicals at Bhopal that is reported to have killed over 8000 people.
- The Chernobyl nuclear power station accident, according to a report prepared by the International Atomic Energy Agency and the World Health Organization, caused 56 deaths directly and caused at least 4000 extra cancer cases.
- The world's worst airliner accident at Tenerife in 1977 claimed 583 lives.
- The explosion on the Piper Alpha oil rig in the North Sea in July 1988 killed 167 workers and completely destroyed the £1 billion oil rig.
- Exxon spent an estimated $2 billion cleaning up after the oil spill when its tanker Exxon Valdez ran aground off the Alaskan coast, and spent a further $1 billion to settle related civil and criminal charges.

The consequences of accidents can even threaten the very existence of an organization. There have been cases where the financial or legal consequences of a catastrophe have forced the organization to close down, be taken over by competing companies or to dismiss their entire senior management team. The Hatfield rail disaster led to the closure of the private company, Railtrack, and the take-over of its assets by the nationalized organization Network Rail.

The impact of nuclear accidents has had a profound effect on the public's perception of the viability of the nuclear power industry. The workforce in the nuclear power industry anticipate that another major nuclear accident anywhere in the world could create such a level of public resistance to nuclear power that the very future of the industry could be jeopardized. Everyone could lose their jobs!

The Corporate Manslaughter and Corporate Homicide Act (see below), which came into force in the UK in April 2008, has created a new criminal offence. When an organization's activities cause a person's death and where the standards of the organization's safety procedures fall far below what can reasonably be expected of the organization in the circumstances, that organization may now be criminally liable. The impact on an organization's reputation of such a charge (let alone conviction) is seen as being very negative.

Thus in safety-critical organizations, the avoidance of adverse events is of primary importance. It not only serves to ensure profits are not wiped out by the costs of accidents, but also ensures public confidence in the ability of organizations to maintain a good safety record. Many HROs regard attention to safety as way of safeguarding public confidence and of safeguarding profit.

The Corporate Manslaughter and Corporate Homicide Act 2007

In the UK, the great majority of clinical negligence cases against NHS Hospital Trusts are brought under *civil* law. In the case of hospital practice, a doctor (or more specifically under vicarious liability his employer—usually a hospital trust) is liable for damages, under civil law, if he is in breach of his duty of care (i.e. if the care he has given was substandard) and if that breach has led to harm to a patient.

Where a doctor commits a *gross* breach of duty and a patient dies as a consequence of this, the doctor is liable for manslaughter under the *criminal* law. This allows the imposition of a custodial sentence on the doctor. A gross breach is conduct that falls *far* below what can be reasonably expected of the doctor in the circumstances. It falls to a jury to define when conduct is far below that expected.

In some cases, systems failures within the healthcare organization, rather than individual doctors, are the root cause for the patient's death. For example, in the Southampton case, the hospital failed to provide an adequate system for supervision of junior doctors over weekends. No senior doctor did ward rounds at weekends. The junior doctors were essentially left to look after patients on the wards on their own. As a consequence, two junior doctors failed to make a diagnosis of septicaemia in a young man who had undergone a routine operation on his knee. The patient subsequently died from septicaemic shock. Failure to make the diagnosis and institute appropriate treatment amounted to gross negligence.

The enactment of the Corporate Manslaughter and Corporate Homicide Act 2007, which came into force in April 2008, creates a new statutory offence of corporate manslaughter (or 'corporate homicide' in Scotland). It provides for an organization to be found liable for failings that led to the death of a patient. The Act removes the key obstacle to convicting large organizations, namely the need to convict the directing mind of the organization. Now senior managers, lower in seniority than the head of the organization, can be found to be liable for the failings of the organization. 'Senior' managers are those who are responsible for the organization and running of the services provided by a hospital and can include hospital managers, doctors, or senior nurses with management responsibilities.

If convicted, the organization can face an unlimited fine. Added to this, the adverse publicity involved in a prosecution is seen as having significant deterrent value. The offences under the Act only cover organizations; there is no individual offence and no one can be sent to prison. However, the common law offence of individual gross negligence manslaughter still exists, allowing convicted individuals to be sentenced to up to life imprisonment.

In the case of hospitals, the Act will hopefully focus the minds of senior management (including doctors with senior managerial roles) on their responsibilities with regard to patient safety. Those duties and responsibilities remain the same, but the consequences of failure to carry out those duties and responsibilities are now substantially more serious for the organization than before.

'Convergent evolution' and its implication for healthcare

The achievements of the HROs would not be quite so interesting had they all merely 'imported' the safety culture and practices of one particular industry and copied them. In biological terms their independent but similar solutions to hazard and risk is an example of 'convergent evolution'—the process by which organisms of different evolutionary origins, when subjected to similar conditions and pressures, have a tendency to develop similar adaptive mechanisms.

Although the various HROs are quite different to each other in many ways, they seem to have *independently* evolved very similar safety cultures. HROs have tried different solutions to their differing human error issues. They have discarded ideas that do not work and developed those that have shown promise.

Therefore, when healthcare looks for ideas to enhance patient safety, they will find in the 'high-reliability' approach a system of measures that have been proven to be effective in a number of widely differing domains. Thus there would seem to be a strong underlying logic in the HRO approach that commends itself for serious consideration as a model for healthcare.

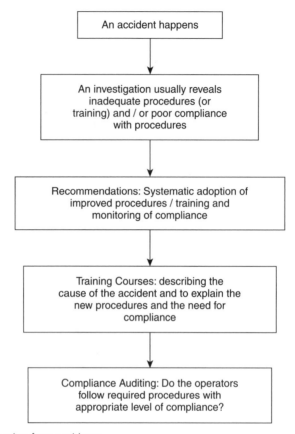

Fig. 3.1 Learning from accidents.

Learning from accidents: overview of basic high reliability organizational culture

The HRO culture is driven by accidents and the need to learn from them (Fig. 3.1).

Elements of the safety culture

Investigation of accidents/near misses

Major accidents can have a profound effect on HROs. An investigation will, in almost all cases, be carried out by an outside agency. Such agencies will have considerable experience in the investigation of adverse events and in creating recommendations for workable and effective remedies.

In most cases the immediate cause of the accident is found to be human error. However, the investigation will search for the 'root causes', which induced this error. In the very rare case where there was gross incompetence by the employee concerned, the investigation focuses on how the employee's incompetence was not detected by the organization's revalidation procedures. If a general fecklessness among operational staff is found then immediate measures would be taken to instil safer behaviours.

In the majority of cases the investigation report usually recommends improvements to be made to the organization's procedures. Reports of accident and incident investigations are freely available to the entire industry.

HRO's recognize that they are at risk from accident scenarios that had not previously occurred. Existing procedures may not offer protection from such problems. These 'new' types of adverse event may be induced by new technologies or changes in the operational environment. Thus in advanced HRO safety cultures, organizations will proactively analyse their 'near miss' incident data to predict and prevent accident scenarios that have not happened yet.

There are currently no independent adverse event investigation agencies in healthcare.

Hospital personnel with little training or experience in human factors or familiarity with HRO concepts often have to carry out investigations.

Reports of their investigations are frequently withheld or at the very least not widely distributed throughout the organization or health service as a whole. The excuse of maintaining 'patient confidentiality' is often given. As a result the wider audience of healthcare workers fails to learn the lessons of accidents and the same type of adverse events recur repeatedly.

Standard operating procedures

In the 1840s the first railway rule books were created in order to prevent accidents. It was said these rule books were 'written in blood', the rules being based on the lessons learned in accidents. In the 1960s a 'before take-off checklist' for pilots was published and against each item on the list was noted the date and location of the accident that had resulted from a pilots' failure to check that particular item before take-off.

In most cases it was obvious which potential error the procedure was designed to prevent. Where the connection was less obvious, an explanation was given.

Thus safety-critical operations in HROs are carried out in accordance with carefully designed standard operating procedures. These procedures include the use of checklists, briefings, announcements, standardized techniques, sequences of actions, and the use of standard communication protocols. Rigid rules (red rules) prevent activities from being carried out if safe conditions or serviceable equipment are not available.

Unusual or abnormal conditions frequently arise during operations in HROs and employees are trained how to depart safely from the standard procedures when necessary. The team leader is required to announce why and how a non-standard procedure is to be used.

Standard procedures specify standard sequences of actions and these standard sequences of actions minimize error during handovers between teams and shifts. This is because it is simpler to describe to the new team or shift which step of the standard procedure has been reached. For the same reason it allows a safe resumption of work after interruptions and substitutions between team members.

Standard operating procedures facilitate the rapid detection of errors. Studies of accidents show that departures from standard procedures often define the moment that the final stage of an accident scenario begins. Team members are required to question why there has been a departure from the standard procedure.

Many healthcare professionals suggest that it is inappropriate to apply the rigid standard operating procedures that are used in HROs to healthcare given the wide range of scenarios encountered in clinical practice (they argue that healthcare 'operations' are too diverse).

Procedures adopted after an adverse event in a hospital are often only applied *locally* rather than system-wide and yet the same event could occur in other locations. In one hospital a fatal patient misidentification error occurred after two patients with similar names were admitted to the same ward. A simple but effective protocol was created to highlight the presence of two patients with similar names. However, this was only applied in the ward where the incident had occurred, with the ward across the corridor not using it even though the same type of error could occur there just as easily!

Culture of confidence and trust: 'fair blame' culture

HROs encourage their staff to have confidence in the efficacy of their error management systems. If people do not believe that checklists and standard operating systems will work reliably they may not use them with sufficient diligence.

Operators must be able to trust that the management will not deal with them harshly when they admit to their errors. In HROs errors are generally not assumed to be moral failures. There is a 'fair blame' culture.

In contrast, in healthcare, it has been suggested that there is a 'culture of low expectations'.

The term 'culture of low expectations' was devised by Mark Chassin and Elise Becher. They described a patient mix-up case where the wrong patient was subjected to an invasive cardiac procedure at an American hospital. Throughout the preparations for the procedure about a dozen 'red flags' were encountered (such as the absence of data about heart problems in the wrong patient's file). However, nothing was done to resolve the problem.

When a system routinely produces error-inducing situations (missing paperwork, miscommunications between team members, changes of plan), clinicians become inured to poorly functioning systems. In such a system, events that should be regarded as red flags—as a major warning of impending danger—are ignored as *normal* operating conditions.

Sociologists have a term: 'learned helplessness', which describes the behaviours and attitudes of a group of people who are living in such an unsatisfactory situation (the term 'learned' indicates that the behaviours and the attitudes are not instinctive but are induced by the cultural environment). People in such a culture come to believe that there is nothing they can do to change things for the better. This then becomes a self-perpetuating situation. Nothing changes because no one makes it change.

The culture of 'low expectations' and the culture of 'learned helplessness' can be successfully challenged with human factors training and other initiatives. This training can show that other domains have addressed similar problems successfully. 'High reliability' can be achieved.

Training

Technical skills training

As one would expect HROs provide a high standard of technical skills training and training in how to carry out their work within the standard operating procedures framework.

Human factors training

In addition, HROs provide employees with a programme of 'non-technical skills training'. These skills include error management, teamwork, and communication protocols for use in safety-critical situations. These skills ensure that operators work effectively within teams working in high-risk situations.

On the training courses a series of accident case studies are analysed and compared. Delegates are encouraged to reflect on their own attitudes and behaviours. The notion that 'it could not happen to me' is challenged. Employees are informed of the theory of HRO and their own responsibilities in such a culture. Duties include reporting your own errors so that the system can be aware of all error-inducing conditions.

Induction training

New employees joining a department in an HRO are given full and detailed instructions on exactly how to carry out their work. The limits of their competence and duties are clearly defined. Specific error-inducing situations that arise in that department's work are described. Employees are given exact instructions on what to do if they encounter uncertainty in their work.

> Healthcare does not, as a general rule, provide 'non-technical skills training' or adequate induction training to clinicians. The results of the latter omission are seen in the cases where junior doctors make errors when they work outside their areas of competence.

Personnel and process auditing

It is not enough for management to lay down procedures and then assume they will be followed. HROs actively monitor the workforce's compliance with required standards. If standards are not being followed it may be because the procedure is unworkable or they have not won the hearts and minds of the workforce to follow the procedures. The performance of individual employees is periodically reviewed. Equipment is tested on a regular basis. Emergency drills are carried out. Follow-ups on problems revealed in periodic audits are an important element.

> Politically driven performance targets in the NHS and staffing levels that are barely adequate for running a clinical service, mean that staff have no time to take 'time outs' to review safety procedures or the efficiency of healthcare processes.

Risk consciousness

A HRO acknowledges the 'high-risk' nature of its activities. Moreover it recognizes that sometimes there are conditions in the working environment that can be deceptively dangerous. Thus, it is inevitable that situations are created during normal operations, which may induce their operators to make the wrong mental model and thus make an error. Consequently, errors and equipment failures are expected to happen at all times. Personnel are trained to 'stop and think' before they carry out non-routine actions. At critical points in procedures in high-risk operations, operators assume the worst case—for example, that every safety-critical communication will be misunderstood.

> The chief medical officer Professor Sir Liam Donaldson has called for the creation of a 'risk-conscious' culture in the NHS to help reduce the rate of adverse events.

Open management/balanced hierarchy

In open management teams juniors are allowed to speak up. This, however, has to be carefully balanced with the need for team leaders to assert their authority. Management encourages and rewards open communication from top to bottom within the organization and ensures that there is collaboration from all ranks to seek solutions to safety problems.

HROs make sure decisions are made at the lowest level commensurate with the problem. The individual who has the highest level of awareness of the operational situation at the front line and the most expertise makes the decisions, not the person of highest rank. This is termed 'migrating decision-making'. Senior managers do not micro-manage or waste time considering lesser problems. HROs organize themselves with sufficient flexibility to allow them to quickly change their structures in response to changes in their environment.

> The culture of most healthcare organizations discourages juniors from speaking up.

'Redundancy' in hardware, personnel, and procedures

Procedures and equipment are designed with back-up systems. A mislaid document should not cause an unsafe situation. There are spare staff to avoid hazard-inducing changes operational activities when a team member is unavailable. As a result there is excess resource provision so there is the opportunity for taking time out for continuous review and innovation in times of average workload.

> High workloads prevent healthcare staff from having the time to analyse and improve working arrangements. Part of that workload might have been created by errors and inefficiency.

Limitations on production

HROs require their operators to stop activities when critical pieces of equipment are not available or when environmental conditions are unfavourable. Precisely written 'red rules' explicitly prohibit activity under these conditions. This provides a powerful incentive for managers to address those situations where 'red rules' are invoked.

> Doctors feel great reluctance to withhold treatment and stop activities when, for example, the patient's notes are missing.
>
> 'Work-arounds', a common feature of operating conditions in healthcare systems, are frequently associated with adverse events. If doctors were to consistently withhold treatment in this type of situation it is possible that hospital managers would more actively address the situations where these problems arise. While causing inconvenience in the short term, greater good would be achieved in the long term.

Active maintenance of the safety culture

One might think that a HRO safety culture becomes self-sustaining. However, there is evidence that active and continuing management is necessary.

A paediatric intensive care unit in California was set up using, from the outset, a HRO safety culture.[6] After a change of leadership the unit returned to the steep hierarchy culture. Important outcome variables such as infant mortality, patient return to the PICU after discharge, days on the PICU, all degraded.

Training in techniques to avoid human error should not be regarded as a one of process, but as an ongoing, organizational wide programme of training. A helpful analogy is that of painting the Forth Road Bridge—as soon as the job is done, it starts again. Painting (maintaining) the bridge is a constant process.

Counter-intuitive aspects of high reliability organization safety culture

There is a problem when attempting to import ideas from HROs into healthcare. Some ideas from HROs seem, at first sight, to be strange, impractical, unworkable, or excessively time-consuming.

Counter-intuitive aspects of a safety culture include the following.

Procedures that might seem to take extra time may actually save time

Taking a 'time out' before a surgical procedure to carry out checks or a briefing seems to add to the total time that the procedures take. However, it is possible that if faulty equipment, missing test results, or missing equipment are discovered before the procedure starts it might be safer, easier, and quicker to sort out the problem at that time rather than when the procedure is in progress.

If you follow HRO communication protocols and ask someone to repeat back a verbal instruction that you have given them, this might seem to increase the amount of time used to communicate. This practice will actually add, say, 15 seconds to the duration of each communication process.

Consider a possible scenario shown in Table 3.1—adjust these rates of misunderstanding for your own specialty (maybe a failure rate of 2 in 100 is too low), adjust the average time spent tracking down missing results, average time spent dealing with consequences of misunderstanding, etc. Thus extra time spent 'reading back' may well save a greater amount of time at other times and in other places.

Table 3.1 Possible scenario using 'read back'

With no read back	With read back
On 100 occasions you ask a colleague to arrange a test on a patient. You do not ask for read back of your instructions	On 100 occasions you ask a colleague to arrange a test on a patient. You ask for read back of your instruction
On two occasions in a hundred your colleague fails to understand the request and the test is not done	Each read back takes 15 seconds
Subsequently, it takes you an additional 30 minutes on each occasion looking for the test result, then organizing a test when you find that it has not been carried out. This interrupts your planned schedule while you do this and then you have to resume your work. Added to this are the problems arising from delayed treatment of the patient	On two occasions in a hundred a misunderstanding is corrected
Total time wasted 60 minutes (more if an adverse events results)	Total time additional time spent 'reading back' 100 × 15 seconds = 25 minutes

A safety culture produces financial savings by enhancing efficiency

Initial studies of HROs suggested that they would have higher operating cost bases than other types of organization. Certainly high-reliability procedures and taking employees out of the front line for regular safety training would seem to impose additional costs on the organization.

However, 'low-cost' airlines such as EasyJet are, by definition, HROs. They have to operate within very narrow profit margins. They cannot afford to have accidents, and indeed by sticking to rigid safety procedures and practices, they believe that their overall efficiency is enhanced. For example, Southwest Airlines, another 'low-cost' airline in the USA appreciates that situations that cause accidents also cause inefficiency. As a result Southwest Airlines was a leader in developing a new compliance monitoring system: LOSA (Line Operation Safety Audit). This system would, in itself, seem to be relatively costly, requiring the recruitment of additional personnel. However, Southwest Airlines believes that it creates a net saving by reducing adverse events and also reducing operational inefficiencies. The regulatory authorities have been impressed by LOSA and are likely to make the process mandatory within the next few years.[7]

Safety procedures and systems can produce hazards of their own

Safety procedures and systems are not problem-free panaceas. Like any medication, they can have side-effects. James Reason in 'Managing the Risks of Organizational Accidents',[8] described the phenomenon of 'Causing the next accident by trying to prevent the last one'.

One factor that may have contributed to the 1977 Tenerife air disaster was the fact that the crew were running out of duty hours. Following a series of aircraft accidents that were attributed to fatigue, aviation authorities introduced mandatory rules restricting the number of hours pilots could work. Owing to a lengthy delay caused by a terrorist incident earlier in the day, the crew of one of the aircraft had to take off very quickly in order to complete the flight within the maximum number of crew duty hours or risk having to night-stop with large costs in accommodating passengers overnight. In their rush to get airborne they misunderstood an air traffic control instruction. Thus a procedure to prevent crew fatigue accidents undoubtedly caused another accident.

Personnel must be alert to the risks of problems arising from the new procedures and safety systems. In aviation, new checklists and procedures are tested in a simulator before they are used on aircraft carrying fare-paying passengers.

Limited number of error categories

HROs gather data on their errors and accidents. In order to analyse these data, errors and accidents have to be categorized. Although it might seem that there would be an infinite number of ways that people can 'screw up', it is interesting to note that the total number of different types of error that *actually* do occur is surprisingly limited. Although some types of error may be resistant to simple error management measures, many categories of error can be relatively easy to manage. It seems to make sense to address those types of error first. This could release time to address the next tier of problems in an iterative approach.

Focus on failure

Compared with healthcare organizations, HROs appear obsessed by the possibility of failure. The overwhelming majority of the documentation sent to pilots by airline management is safety related. This is mainly to create awareness of error-inducing situations revealed by recent incidents.

> HROs do not necessarily aim for excellence in their operations; they seek merely to avoid failure.

This is a humble aim, perhaps, but one that some of them seem able to achieve with nearly 100% success.

Focus on seemingly trivial details

In studying their disasters, HROs have noted that many began with seemingly trivial misunderstandings and flawed assumptions about issues that appeared to the operators at the time to be irrelevant.

At least one individual in healthcare is aware of this: The distinguished paediatric cardiac surgeon, Professor Marc de Leval discovered that small errors in the operating theatre or during the process of transferring children from the theatre to ITU '... are the most important types of error because they are not even perceived by the team, very little is done to compensate for them and they add to each other and influence very significantly the outcomes.'[9]

Because small errors are perceived not to have an effect on the safety of the system no one attempts to do anything about them. HROs have learned that they do have to attend very closely and in very great detail to some, but not all, aspects of their operations. A 'risk-conscious' culture develops the ability of personnel to assess which trivia they need to attend to and which they can ignore.

Rewarding error (or more correctly the admission of error)

The nature of the safety culture on the aircraft carrier is well illustrated by the following true story.[10] A junior mechanic once lost one of his tools while working on the landing deck. He realized the considerable danger that the item could create if it were sucked into a jet engine or if it jammed in the aircraft launching catapult mechanism. He immediately reported his loss and all activity on the deck was halted while a search was carried out. Aircraft intending to land on the carrier had to be diverted to land bases. Some time later the tool was found. One might have imagined that the mechanic would have been punished for his carelessness. However, the next day there was a formal ceremony to commend the mechanic for his honesty and his courage in admitting to his error.

There is a balance to be struck here. One might think that, in this case, rewarding the mechanic could encourage others to be careless. However, the commanding officers took the view that encouraging honesty was much more important. Punishing the mechanic would almost certainly have led to other errors being concealed.

Error is seen as 'normal'

HROs encourage their personnel to expect error and failure at all times. For example, it becomes instinctive to assume that every safety-critical message will be misunderstood. As a result, personnel insist safety-critical messages are repeated back by recipients.

Application of 'kindergarten' methodologies

One might imagine that the HROs always employ sophisticated technologies to control their operations. This is not necessarily the case.

The US Navy created a complex computer program to plan and execute the movement of aircraft on the crowded deck of their aircraft carriers. They found it difficult to use. It proved to be very difficult to input data on the location of aircraft fast enough for operations to continue at the required pace.

The computerized system was discarded and in its place a simple scale model of the deck was made—literally a table top shaped like the deck of the carrier. Toy aeroplanes were used. The pre-flight preparation status of the aircraft was represented by placing nuts and bolts on top of the toy aeroplanes. Nuts represented the fact that weapons had been loaded and bolts the fact that the aircraft had been refuelled. This simplified the process of determining where each plane was, whether it could move past other parked aircraft, whether it had been refuelled and re-armed, etc.

The system proved to be very simple, very quick, and very reliable, giving the crew in charge of flight deck operations a very good mental model of how flight deck operations were proceeding. In this way the deck operations' officers can see the operational situation at a glance and thus plan efficient movements and operations. As a result error-inducing situations such as changes of plan (when it is found that one aircraft cannot get past another in the confined spaces on the deck, for example) can be minimized.

On the flight deck itself, the deck crews wear colour-coded jackets. Weapons loaders wear red, refuellers blue, and so on. In this way personnel can see at a glance which activities are being carried out on which aircraft on the deck. In this way operational 'situation awareness' is enhanced.

Such systems are incredibly simple and require no sophisticated technology. The US Navy has adopted them because it believes that they enhance safety and efficiency.

Many HROs encourage their personnel to point to critical words in documents, reading them out loud, in a way reminiscent of teaching kindergarten children to read.

'Stating the obvious' is encouraged in some situations in order to eliminate the remote possibility that someone has adopted the wrong mental model.

Reported incidents increase

Accountants will require evidence that training interventions to enhance patient safety are cost-effective. Owing to a culture of under-reporting in organizations with underdeveloped safety cultures, the adoption of a high reliability culture will actually produce an increase in reported incidents. Thus it may be impossible to prove in the short term that patient safety training produces an immediate financial benefit.

References

1 **Weick KE, Sutcliffe KM.** *Managing the unexpected: assuring high performance in an age of complexity*. San Francisco, CA: Jossey-Bass; 2001.

2 **Reason J.** Human error: models and management. *Br Med J* 2000; **320**:768–70.

3 **LaPorte TR.** The United States air traffic control system: increasing reliability in the midst of rapid growth. In: *The development of large technical systems* (eds R Mayntz, TP Hughes). Boulder, CO: Westview Press; 1988.

4 **Roberts KH.** Managing high reliability organizations. *Calif Manage Rev* 1990; **32**: 101–13.

5 **Helmreich R.** On error management: lessons from aviation. *Br Med J* 2000; **320**: 781–5.

6 **Roberts K H, Madsen P, Desai V, Van Stralen D.** A case of the birth and death of a high reliability healthcare organisation. *Qual Saf Health Care* 2005; **14**: 216–20.

7 **Griffith V.** *Safety first*. University of Texas at Austin website http://www.utexas.edu/ features/archive/2004/safety.html/.

8 **Reason J.** *Managing the risks of organizational accidents*. Aldershot: Ashgate Publishing Ltd; 1997.

9 Television interview with Professor Marc de Leval: Channel 4 programme: *Why doctors make mistakes—breaking the code of silence*. Available from Darlow Smithson Productions http://www.darlowsmithson.com/.

10 **Landau M, Chisholm D.** The arrogance of optimism: notes on failure avoidance management. *J Contingencies Crisis Manage* 1995; **3**: 67–80.

Further reading

Bigley GA, Roberts KH. The incident command system: high-reliability organizing for complex and volatile task environments. *Acad Manage J* 2001; **44**: 1281–99.

Grabowski M, Roberts K. Risk mitigation in large-scale systems: lessons from high reliability organizations. *Calif Manage Rev* 1997; **39**: 152–62.

Grabowski M, Roberts KH. Risk mitigation in virtual organizations. *Organ Sci* 1999; **10**: 704–21.

Klein LR, Bigley GA, Roberts KH. Organizational culture in high reliability organizations: an extension. *Hum Relat* 1995; **48**: 771–93.

La Porte TR. High Reliability Organisations: unlikely, demanding, and at risk. *J Contingencies Crisis Manage* 1996; **4**: 60–71.

Roberts KH. Managing high reliability organizations. *Calif Manage Rev* 1990; **32**: 101–13.

Roberts KH. Some characteristics of one type of high reliability organization. *Organ Sci* 1990; **1**: 160–76. [Abstract]

Roberts KH, Bea R. Must accidents happen? Lessons from high-reliability organisations. *Acad Manage Exec* 2001; **15**: 70–8.

Roberts KH, Bea RG. When systems fail. *Organ Dyn* 2001; **29**: 179–87.

Roberts KH, La Porte TR, Rochlin GI. The self-designing high-reliability organization: aircraft carrier flight operations at sea. *Naval War Coll Rev* (reprinted) 1998; 97–113.

Schulman P, Emery R, van Eeten M, de Bruijne M. High reliability and the management of critical infrastructures. *J Contingencies Crisis Manage* 2004; **12**: 14–28.

Weick KE. Organizational culture as a source of high reliability. *Calif Manage Rev* 1987; **29**; 112–27.

Chapter 4

Case studies

Those industries that have successfully reduced their accident rates have done so by creating in their work forces an awareness of the aetiology of adverse events. Fundamental to this is the seemingly mawkish practice of studying in some detail the scenarios of adverse event cases. The narrative of these stories is designed to demonstrate how one might make the same mistake.

The use of case studies is one of the principal vehicles of instruction on safety courses in high reliability organizations. Without case studies these courses can be too theoretical. Case studies add a sense of realism to what can, at times, be a dry subject.

Telling someone to be careful in a particular situation may increase their caution for a while. However, narrating to them, with the appropriate level of detail the circumstances of a real adverse event seems to have a more profound and enduring effect. This has certainly been the experience of the airline industry where pilots listen to real-life recordings of accidents and near misses as recorded on the cockpit voice recorder. Listening to the voice of someone who you know died just a few minutes after their voice was recorded on to tape can be a chilling experience. The lessons learned from studying these recordings have played a major role in preventing recurrences of accidents.

What is striking in many of the recordings is the similar types of dialogue that occur in the 30 minutes prior to a crash. The dialogue in healthcare errors bears many similarities. If teams of doctors and nurses could be heard speaking on hospital black box recorders, common themes that lead to errors would emerge—loss of situation awareness through the stress of an evolving disaster, poorly worded messages, failure to speak up, etc.

With this in mind we have *deliberately* discussed three examples of wrong-sided surgery (all nephrectomies) and three examples of intrathecal vincristine injections. This is not because of a poverty of ideas on our behalf, but rather because all of these cases demonstrate the recurring nature of error. The three intrathecal vincristine scenarios all began differently, but they all ended up progressing along common error pathways with the final outcome being the same in each case: an inexperienced doctor sitting behind a young man's back with a syringe full of vincristine, unwittingly about to kill the patient. In the words of Tony Barrell, a safety expert who assisted Lord Cullen in the Piper Alpha Oil Platform Inquiry: 'There is an awful sameness about these incidents. They are nearly always characterised by lack of forethought and lack of analysis, and nearly always the problem comes down to poor management.'

This perfectly sums up why the Great Ormond Street vincristine error was followed by the same error at Queen's Medical Centre in Nottingham.

Thus, these cases demonstrate that the same old errors keep cropping up—with frightening or boring regularity (however you care to look at it)! They demonstrate that these errors are not one-off events. They represent fundamental aspects of aberrant human psychology and behaviour working in combination with poorly designed systems. This provides the perfect conditions for inducing error, where error preventing strategies are not in operation.

We hope that any repetition in the cases described will not bore the reader, but rather will reinforce the important messages contained in these sad stories. We must also say that it is not our intention that this collection of case studies be seen as a representative sample of *all* adverse events, but we hope that those described do contain some useful lessons of why errors can occur and how they might be prevented.

The selection and presentation of the case studies requires careful consideration. While useful lessons can be learned from almost all adverse events, a number of case studies will be particularly instructive and memorable. This might be because of the time or location of their occurrence, the dramatic nature of the scenario or something someone said such as 'Aren't you taking out the wrong kidney?'

Preventability

Errors can be classified in a variety of different ways. One important classification is how preventable they are. Clearly, some types of error are easier to prevent than others. Organizations that initiate error management programmes invariably target the most preventable errors first before addressing the more difficult types of error.

> There is a powerful logic to the argument that if you cannot stop the most preventable errors from happening, then you will certainly have trouble preventing the harder ones

Wrong side surgery and medication errors are generally easier to prevent than, say, the diagnostic errors that can occur when dealing with patients with highly atypical symptoms. Thus, the case studies on the following pages start with a number of highly preventable adverse events.

In other safety critical industries, the most catastrophic, highly preventable disasters, such as the Tenerife air disaster, the Piper Alpha Oilrig explosion, and Chernobyl, have led to major beneficial changes in organization, although these accidents were not typical (in terms of their enormity) of the types of adverse event that normally occur.

It can be seen that most of the case studies in this chapter result from error chains that could have been easily broken at any point along the way, but for the want of an understanding of how errors can occur and of preventative techniques. Subsequent chapters in this book demonstrate that the *individual* healthcare worker may be the only one capable of breaking the chain. That so much hinges on the actions of an individual might seem a frightening prospect, but the other more optimistic side of the coin is that the *individual* can have such a dramatic and positive effect on error reduction—if he or she knows the simple tools that allow error chains to be broken.

Case study 1: wrong patient

During a patient safety course at a hospital in London delegates were asked to describe any instructive adverse events with which they were involved. One delegate, a medical registrar, described how he had made a fatal error some years earlier. While in the middle of a busy outpatient clinic, he was asked to go to a ward to carry out a liver biopsy on a Mrs K.

It was necessary to deliver the sample before the path lab closed at 4.30 that Friday afternoon. He telephoned the ward in advance to ask that the trolley with the necessary equipment be placed by the patient's bedside ready for him. Breathless from his run up four flights of stairs, he arrived at the nurse's station. He was told that Mrs K was the 'lovely little old lady in the bed by the window at the far end of the ward'.

He arrived at the bed and saw Mrs K's name over the bed. He greeted her: 'Mrs K?' The patient replied: 'Hello Doctor'. He had the correct patient—he thought. He carried out the biopsy under local anaesthesia.

The following morning the patient was found dead.

It turned out that patient from whom he had taken the sample was another patient who suffered with senile dementia and in her chronic confusional state she had happened to get into the wrong bed while the real Mrs K was away from the ward. This patient suffered from a clotting disorder and during the night bled to death from the site of the liver biopsy.

Comment

In this case the principal 'operator error' was the doctor's failure to actively identify the patient.

This error was, in turn, largely the result of the failure of the hospital (the system) to provide the doctor with training in the 'active identification' of patients. The hospital did not provide patient safety training, which should have included reminders (*regular* reminders) of the importance of consistently checking patient identity before *any* interaction with a patient who you have never met before, whether taking a simple history, prescribing a drug, taking blood, giving a blood transfusion, or performing any procedure, such as a liver biopsy or an operation.

'Active identification' is where the patient is asked to state his or her name. Complete confirmation is obtained when the patient is asked to give their date of birth and/or address. The name, date of birth, and address are then checked against the documentation. ('Passive identification' would be where you ask someone if they are Mrs K or whatever, the only confirmation of this being 'yes or no'.) Remember, a substantial proportion of particularly elderly patients are hard of hearing. It is possible that the bogus Mrs K in the case described above did not hear the name that the doctor said, and simply said 'yes'.

Case study 2: wrong blood

A non-urgent abdominal aortic aneurysm repair in a 64-year-old man was scheduled for 8.30 on a Thursday morning in operating theatre 1 at a hospital in the north of England. The surgical team were led to believe that they would be the only surgical team carrying out surgery at that early hour. The theatre suite was seemingly deserted. A list showed that the first procedure scheduled for the adjoining theatre 2 was a prostatectomy at 10.30 a.m.

The circulating nurse telephoned the blood bank and was assured that the cross-matched units of blood had left the blood bank a moment ago and would be placed in the theatre refrigerator outside the theatre within a minute or two.

Unknown to the surgical team in theatre 1, there had been a change of plan and an additional prostatectomy case had been arranged for theatre 2 at 9.00 a.m. Several units of blood had also been ordered for this patient.

During the operation in theatre 1, the surgeon requested that preparations for a blood transfusion be made. The tone of his voice inadvertently suggested urgency, although there was no particular urgency as there was no significant blood loss at that time.

Owing to the suggested urgency the circulating nurse hurried to the blood refrigerator. She picked the only units that she could see, assuming that it was for her patient, and signed for the blood. She returned to theatre 1 and handed the blood to the anaesthetist.

The anaesthetist knew that the nurse was very conscientious having seen her on many occasions carefully checking the labels on blood units and he presumed that she had checked the blood when she was outside. Because of this the anaesthetist did not check the label himself and immediately started the transfusion.

A few minutes later a nurse from the surgical team in theatre 2 went to the blood refrigerator looking for the blood for her patient. The blood wasn't there even though she had seen it there a few minutes earlier. The blood for the aneurysm repair was there, however. She correctly deduced that the blood for theatre 2 might have been removed in error to be given to the patient in theatre 1. She rushed to the other theatre but it was too late. By this time 100 ml of the wrong blood had already been transfused. The patient who had been given the wrong blood subsequently died as a consequence of a transfusion reaction.

Comment

Why bother to check something (units of blood to be transfused, a patient's name, a drug to be administered) if you are absolutely certain that it is the right one and there is no possibility of the wrong one being there?

This case provides the antidote to such thoughts. A change of plan and a malevolent coincidence can mean that a situation that you think is absolutely certain is really lethally deceptive.

The lesson to learn is that you should never assume that the unit of blood in your hands is the correct one, or that the patient in front of you is the correct one or that the drug you are about to administer is the right one. Nor should you assume that someone else has checked correctly.

Case study 3: wrong side nephrectomy

Mr D, the consultant urological surgeon involved in this case, was well known for his very meticulous and professional manner.

As we see in other safety critical industries, the extremely conscientious and competent operator creates a perverse consequence; colleagues cannot imagine them making a mistake and therefore they do not check them effectively. If they make an error, colleagues cannot believe it and think that they themselves are at fault.

Mr D saw an elderly male patient, with a history of haematuria, in his outpatient clinic. An intravenous urogram (IVU) had been done that afternoon. The films had been returned to the clinic with the patient, but as yet remained unreported. Urine cytology was positive for transitional cell cancer cells.

Mr D looked at the images, several of which demonstrated a filling defect which was highly suggestive of a transitional cell cancer. The image which demonstrated the tumour most clearly had an 'R' (for 'right') on the same side as the filling defect. This led the consultant to the conclusion that this was a right sided tumour. The consultant made a record in the patient's notes "for right nephroureterectomy".

Unfortunately, this *one* image had been incorrectly labelled with a letter 'R' rather than an 'L'. The other images in the IVU series had (correctly) labelled the tumour side as 'L' – a left sided tumour.

When the radiologist's report arrived a few days later it did give the correct side for the tumour (the left). However, the consultant only scanned the report and having created a mental model that the tumour was in the right kidney, he proceeded to carry out a right nephroureterectomy. The procedure was carried out with the high degree of technical skill that the consultant's colleagues had come to expect of him. Blood loss was minimal. There was not associated lymphadenopathy and the consultant anticipated that he had probably cured the patient of his disease.

At the end of the operation the registrar bivalved the kidney, but to his surprise he could find no evidence of a tumor. The consultant was devastated by the error and confessed the mistake to the patient and his family. The patient subsequently underwent a left nephroureterctomy and became dialysis dependent.

Comment

When the patient was prepared for surgery in the operating theatre, no one checked the radiologist's report. No formal verbalized checks were carried out and there was no cross-checking of X-ray film with the radiologist's report. The patient's side was not marked.

The hospital had a general requirement for personnel to make checks but gave no precise guidance as to how this was to be done. There was no auditing to confirm that it was being done.

Case study 4: another wrong side nephrectomy[1,2]

This case received widespread media coverage (and sadly with the usual media approach to error 'analysis'—that of naming, blaming, and shaming—rather than a thoughtful process designed to prevent recurrences of the error).

On a Friday in the year 2000 Mr S a 70-year-old male patient was admitted for a right nephrectomy. The ward had a policy of not writing the 'side' (left kidney or right kidney) on their paperwork. The intention behind this rule was that it would oblige clinicians to check the patient's notes. Using the notes, a junior doctor correctly consented the patient for a right simple nephrectomy for a non-functioning kidney containing stones.

In the afternoon the operation had to be cancelled due to lack of an ITU bed. Remembering that Monday's operating list was probably being prepared at that time, an SHO rushed to the office where the secretary was typing the list. Unfortunately, he did not take any of the patient's paperwork with him and he made a memory error by telling her that the patient required a left nephrectomy.

On the following Monday morning the patient was re-admitted. Knowing that a consent form had been signed on the Friday, staff went ahead with administering the pre-med. Later it was realized that Friday's consent form could not be found and a new consent form was prepared.

Referring to the erroneous operating list, a junior doctor again consented the patient, who was by now somewhat drowsy from his pre-med, for a left nephrectomy. Nurses on the ward were unable to detect this error, as their paperwork did not give the 'side'. Thus the decision not to give the 'side', which was intended to be an error prevention measure, had the unfortunate effect of inhibiting error detection.

The patient was taken to the anaesthetic room with his notes. The consultant, registrar, and medical student entered the operating theatre. The side was not marked as the rule was seen as counterproductive. The consultant saw the operating list and seemed to remember that the patient needed a right nephrectomy.

He was heard to say, 'It's the right isn't it?'. Unfortunately, for some reason the theatre staff were emphatic that the operating list was correct. The consultant said, 'The notes are where you will find the answer!' He went into the anaesthetic room to check the notes.

The anaesthetist was known to firmly discourage visits to the anaesthetic room while he was anaesthetising the patient. The consultant did not seem to be able to ask the anaesthetist to pass the patient's notes, in order to check which kidney was to be removed.

He did look at the admission card, which was on the table near the door. In spite of the apparent confusion, it appears he did not carry out a full check of the notes. At this point he seems to have changed his mind. He returned to the operating theatre but did not say that he had not actually examined the notes. His silence was taken by the theatre staff as a tacit admission that he was wrong about the 'side' for the procedure.

He went to the light box and examined the X-rays with a medical student. Unfortunately, the X-ray film had been placed the wrong way round. For some reason the medical student queried the orientation of the film but was reassured by the consultant.

The registrar asked if he could do the operation with the assistance of the SHO. The operation would be supervised by the consultant who would remain unscrubbed. The registrar was delayed attending to the previous patient on the operating list and arrived about 10 minutes late in theatre to find the patient already draped on the operating table.

The registrar did not examine the hospital notes or check the X-rays. He assumed that the consultant had carried out all of the necessary checks. He was aware that there had been confusion about the correct side for the procedure but this had apparently been resolved by the consultant. During the subsequent investigation he made it clear that he regarded himself as a technician and that he always deferred to the opinion of his chief.

He scrubbed up and made the first incision, unaware that he was operating on the wrong side. The registrar had asked the consultant if he could perform a radical nephrectomy, that is remove the kidney with its envelope of fatty tissue intact. This would normally be the procedure for renal cancer. For benign disease the usual procedure would be to remove the kidney within its investing fascia. Carrying out a radical nephrectomy denied the registrar of the opportunity to see the kidney itself and confirm he was operating on an unhealthy kidney.

During the procedure he had to ligate a healthy pulsating artery before dividing the vessel. In the clinic some days earlier he had discussed with the consultant the presence of a reduced arterial flow to the diseased kidney. He seems to have forgotten this when he was actually carrying out the procedure. During the operation a medical student, Miss F, studied the X-ray. She noticed the apparent difference in the arterial supply to the two kidneys.

She saw the registrar placing a clamp across a powerfully pulsating artery and said she thought it must be supplying the healthy kidney. The X-ray showed a poor supply to the diseased kidney. She told the registrar that she thought that he was operating on the wrong kidney. She was not given the opportunity to explain the evidence behind her comment before the registrar cut her short. He told her that she 'had got it wrong'.

Once excised the kidney was placed in formalin. Postoperatively, it was soon noticed that the patient had a very poor urine output, and only at this point was the mistake detected. The patient died a month later.

The consultant and the registrar were charged with manslaughter but were found not guilty as it was not clear that the wrong-side operation had killed Mr S. The patient had had a pre-existing heart condition.

Comment

As in case study 3, there was inadequate pre-operative checking for similar systemic reasons. There was also a change of plan (the day of the operation changed from Friday to Monday) and an important communication failure (the consultant failed to communicate the result of his checking of the notes in the anaesthetic room). The rejection of the valid input from the medical student was a very noteworthy feature of this case.

Case study 5: yet another wrong side nephrectomy case

Mrs D, aged 55, had had her left kidney removed in 1994. She subsequently devloped renal failure.

In 1995 a transplanted kidney was placed in the lower right iliac fossa, giving her two 'right' kidneys. Initially, this transplanted kidney had not functioned very well but, subsequently, it had established satisfactory function. The patient was admitted to a hospital in 2003 for the removal of her right native kidney, which had become diseased. The operation was listed as 'nephrectomy' followed by a two-letter abbreviation.

This was not a recognized abbreviation for 'right native'. On the day before the operation a keen young urology SHO studied the operating list and noticed this unfamiliar abbreviation.

He asked several colleagues what the abbreviation meant but no one else recognized the abbreviation. He then studied the patient's notes in order to try to understand its meaning. It is possible that at some point the notes may have spilled out of their folder and had been reinserted in the wrong order. The result was that the reports about the initial poor performance of the transplanted kidney were the first pages to be seen on opening the folder.

More careful analysis of later pages in the notes revealed the report about the satisfactory function of the transplanted kidney. The SHO began to realize that it was possible that the surgeon might not understand the meaning of the abbreviation and, after a brief review of the file, might be misled by the initial report about the transplanted kidney. He described his fears about the potential for the removal of the wrong kidney to several colleagues. He did not, however, tell any of the urology consultants, although he did pass one later that afternoon in the corridor.

As the operation was planned to start at 3 p.m. the following afternoon the SHO intended to go to theatres at that time and talk to the surgeon. When he arrived in theatres he found that the operation had already been carried out, having been rescheduled to 1 p.m. The error that he had predicted had been made.

The patient was judged not suitable for a further kidney transplant and the Trust involved is now obliged to pay for the patient's dialysis for the rest of her life.

Comment

This is another example of a checking failure.

In hindsight, it might have been helpful if the SHO had placed a 'post-it' note inside the file in a prominent place drawing attention to the potential confusion and suggesting that a careful review of the notes might be wise. He might have reorganized the file into the correct order. Alternatively he could have personally expressed his concerns to the relevant consultant.

Case study 6: medication error—wrong route (intrathecal vincristine)

Patient T, aged 16, suffered from leukaemia. He came regularly for treatment with cytotoxic drugs at a large general hospital in the South East of England. On a Wednesday in 1990, he was due to have injections of *intravenous* **vincristine** and *intrathecal* **methotrexate**.

The previous day the consultant had filled out the necessary prescription forms on the patient's drugs' chart. He sent them to the pharmacy department for the injections to be prepared. The drugs were duly prepared by the pharmacy and taken to the ward that Patient T was due to attend. They were put in a red box bearing labels indicating that they were cytotoxic drugs. Also on the outside of the box were two labels bearing the patient's name, the name of the drug, and the route by which it was to be injected, that is bearing either the letters 'I.T.' (intrathecal) or 'I.V.' (intravenous).

Inside the box were the two syringes containing the drugs. They too bore labels with the same information upon each of them as the labels on the outside of the box.

On the Tuesday the consultant's secretary realized that only Dr P, an SHO, would be available to give Patient T his lumbar puncture on the next day. She said to him 'Patient T would be coming in at 9.30 am'. From this piece of data she intended that Dr P should infer that he would be giving the injection. However, she did not state this and Dr P was unaware that he would be doing the lumbar puncture and administering the drugs.

On the Wednesday morning the box of cytotoxic drugs was put out on a trolley in the ward. Normally cytotoxic drugs were put on a special cytotoxic trolley to which the pharmaceutical company's data sheet was attached. This data sheet stated that injecting vincristine intrathecally 'can be fatal'.

On this occasion the lumbar-puncture trolley was used because it was larger and could hold all the necessary equipment. Unfortunately, the data sheet, with its warning about vincristine was not transferred from the cytotoxic to the lumbar-puncture trolley.

At about 9.30 a.m. patient T and his mother arrived at the ward. Dr P told them that he did not know if he would be dealing with the matter, as he was inexperienced. He then saw the registrar, Dr C and told him that Patient T had come in for his cytotoxic injections and added that he was reluctant to administer the injections because of his inexperience.

Dr C asked Dr P to get Dr S, another doctor, to supervise him, but added that if Dr S had not done a lumbar puncture previously he (Dr C) would supervise the treatment himself! Dr S had only once previously attempted to do a lumbar puncture and that attempt had failed. He had some limited previous experience of cytotoxic drugs but on only one occasion previously he had injected vincristine intravenously.

A ward sister saw Dr P with Dr S. Dr P made known to her his concern about doing the lumbar puncture. Dr S agreed to supervise. The sister believed that Dr S was going to supervise Dr P during the whole process of doing the lumbar puncture.

But here it appears that a regrettable misunderstanding took place. Dr P thought Dr S was supervising him during the whole procedure, including the checking of, and the administration of the cytotoxic drugs. However, Dr S thought he was there only to supervise the initial placement of the lumbar puncture needle. Dr S thought that he had no responsibility over the administration of the cytotoxic drugs.

Mrs H, an experienced oncology nurse, set up the trolley ready for the lumbar puncture and took this trolley and the red box with the drugs to the side ward where the patient and the two doctors were.

Mrs H had studied information about vincristine and had noted its extremely toxic properties. Some weeks earlier she had discussed with the consultant that the only route for the injection of vincristine was the intravenous one. It was obvious to her that any other route would be extremely harmful. However, in the subsequent manslaughter trial it was revealed that even the consultant was unaware that intrathecal administration of vincristine was always a fatal and irreversible error.

As it happened there were two student nurses on the ward who wished to watch the lumbar puncture. Seeing that there were two doctors and two student nurses present, Mrs H left. In view of the misunderstanding between Dr P and Dr S, this was unfortunate. The two student nurses had no experience of cytotoxic drugs and, as students, were not allowed even to touch them.

Before the lumbar puncture Dr P administered a local anaesthetic. One of the student nurses handed him the local anaesthetic, reading aloud its name in accordance with her training as she did so. After that had been done, Dr P inserted the lumbar puncture needle into the spine successfully. A little CSF leaked out which appeared to trouble Dr P.

He then asked for a pair of goggles, which was the normal procedure when dealing with cytotoxic drugs. After putting them on, he asked for the drugs themselves.

Dr S was not scrubbed up, nor was he wearing gloves. He opened the red box, took out the first syringe and handed it to Dr P. He warned Dr P that the syringe was now not sterile.

This piece of 'data' was undoubtedly true, but what was Dr S's point in saying it? What did Dr S expect Dr P to do? It seemed that Dr P was being asked to give an unsterile injection. This communication seemed to confuse and distract Dr P at a time when he should have been focusing on making checks on the medication.

Dr P then fitted the syringe on to the needle and injected it into the patient's spine. He then unscrewed that syringe and took the second syringe from Dr S and also injected that into the spine. Neither doctor checked the labels on the box or the labels on the syringes before these two injections.

Dr P then went to the preparation room and looked at the data chart on the cytotoxic trolley. He was extremely upset and said: 'Oh my God. It can be fatal.'

Patient T died 4 days later. Both Dr S and Dr P were subsequently found guilty of manslaughter.

On appeal, both convictions were quashed. At the appeal hearing it was noted that Dr P was required to give the treatment without the consultant who prescribed it giving any instruction or thought as to who should do so. This, despite the fact that Dr P was inexperienced, reluctant to give the treatment, and wholly unaware of the likely fatal consequences of giving vincristine by lumbar puncture. Dr P did not have the data chart on the cytotoxic trolley because that trolley was not in use.

The senior nurse was not present, leaving only two students at the scene. Moreover, having asked for supervision and believing that Dr S was supervising the whole treatment, Dr P was actually handed each of the two syringes in turn by Dr S and administered the drugs under his very eyes.

So far as Dr S was concerned, he believed he was simply required to supervise the insertion of the lumbar puncture needle by an inexperienced houseman. He understood the drugs were for administration by lumbar puncture. He did not have special experience or knowledge of cytotoxic drugs.

As a result of this and several other identical cases NHS Trusts adopted a number of different protocols to ensure the intrathecal and intravenous chemotherapy drugs are kept separated.

Case study 7: another medication error—wrong route (intrathecal vincristine)[3]

Patient X, a 12-year-old boy with T-cell non-Hodgkin's lymphoma was due to have injections of *intravenous* **vincristine** and *intrathecal* **methotrexate** at Great Ormond Street Hospital—the world's most famous children's hospital. As Patient X was very frightened of spinal injections he was to be given the methotrexate under general anaesthesia.

The hospital had adopted procedures to ensure intrathecal and intravenous drugs could not be mixed up as had happened in case study 6 above. As a result it was forbidden even to have the two types of drug in the same room or for them to be carried together.

However, on the day that Patient X was to undergo treatment the paediatric oncology ward was full and, therefore, he was admitted to a general paediatric ward. Although oncology patients were routinely admitted to general wards, there were no procedures to advise staff of the protocols related to the separation of chemotherapy drugs.

At 06.15 Patient X was allowed by a nurse to eat a biscuit. As a consequence his general anaesthesia had to be delayed for 6 hours. In the oncology department, the documentation (Nurses' Planning Chart, consent forms, etc.) erroneously showed that only one drug, the methotrexate, was to be administered that day. Patient X's medical notes were mislaid until mid-morning so this error could not be detected.

At about 10.00 Dr G, the anaesthetist, visited Patient X and discovered that he had eaten the biscuit and arranged for his general anaesthesia to be delayed. Some of the doctors and nurses were informed of this change; others were not. On one list Patient X was transferred to the afternoon list. At about 10.45 there was a brief discussion between Dr W (the haematology consultant), Dr G, and one other doctor about who was to carry out the procedure on Patient X. Unfortunately at the end of this discussion there was no summing up of the discussion and each person had a different understanding of what they thought they had agreed.

Shortly afterwards, Dr G managed to persuade Patient X to have the intrathecal injection under local anaesthetic. This meant he could still be treated in the morning.

Owing to an oversight in the pharmacy the two drugs were sent *together* to the ward. The nurses in the general paediatric ward had not been trained to recognize the danger of this. They did, however, note the extreme danger associated with vincristine.

At 11.40 Patient X was taken to the theatre along with the two drugs. It now seemed that it would be left to Dr G to give the medication. This anaesthetic registrar had never given intrathecal cytotoxic treatment before and was somewhat uneasy about doing this.

He discussed this procedure by telephone with the haematology consultant, Dr W, who reassured him that it was a simple procedure. Dr W had seen the list showing only methotrexate was to be administered that day and expected therefore only methotrexate to be present in theatre. Therefore, Dr W told him to inject the drug (singular) intrathecally, which the pharmacy had sent up. Dr G did not tell him that two syringes (plural) had been sent up. Neither party mentioned the name of the drug/drugs.

The hand-written documents supplied by the pharmacy department had abbreviated intrathecal to 'it' and intravenous to 'iv' (lower case). Dr G did not notice this important distinction.

A nurse provided Dr G with two syringes, one containing vincristine and bearing a label that read 'only for iv use'. The nurse noticed that Dr G was not wearing any gloves when administering the drugs. The consultants had always been very careful to put their gloves on before handling vincristine. The nurse did not speak up and point this out to the doctor. If she had done this, the extreme danger associated with vincristine might have been drawn to his attention.

Dr G correctly injected the methotrexate into the spine. He then incorrectly administered the vincristine intrathecally.

Patient X developed an increasingly painful arachnoiditis, which was diagnosed 2 days after the episode. He subsequently died in considerable pain.

In July 2000 the Department of Health published a document entitled *An organization with a memory*,[4] which drew attention to the failure of the NHS to learn from its mistakes. At the press conference to launch the document, Professor Sir Liam Donaldson, the Chief Medical Officer, commented on the previous cases where vincristine had been administered intrathecally and said that the accident must never happen again. Tragically, in spite of seemingly foolproof procedures and the Chief Medical Officer drawing attention to the danger, the error happened again. This case is described below.

Case study 8: medication error—wrong route (intrathecal vincristine)[5,6]

A year after publication of *An organization with a memory* Mr P died at the Queens Medical Centre, Nottingham after vincristine was wrongly injected into his spine. So much for memory!

Mr P was diagnosed with acute lymphoblastic leukaemia in 1999. By June 2000 he was in remission, but still needed 3-monthly injections of two chemotherapeutic agents—vincristine and cytosine. Hospital management had a policy of not giving patients both drugs on the same day.

Mr P's appointment had originally been scheduled just before Christmas but he could not face a painful spinal injection at that time and the appointment was rescheduled for 4 January 2001. Unfortunately, while this date was written into the ward diary, it was not entered into the ward manager's chemotherapy diary. As a result Mr P's chemotherapy was not ordered in advance and Christmas leave prevented this error being detected by staff.

The omission was discovered on the Monday morning and the following order was sent down to pharmacy: cytosine i.t. 4 January 2001 and vincristine i.v. 5 January 2001. He was to receive the cytosine on Monday 4 January and the vincristine the following day. The pharmacist made up the cytosine and the pre-loaded vincristine syringe but wrote the date on both as 4 January 2001. At about 10 a.m. both drugs were sent from the pharmacy to the ward together. They were in similar syringes and both clear liquids and although clearly labelled they were stored together on the ward's fridge.

Mr P arrived in the afternoon for his morning appointment: he had been very worried about the treatment and needed some time to 'psyche' himself up, hence his late attendance. Dr H, the consultant in charge of Mr P's case, was aware that his patient was very late and asked ward staff to tell him when Mr P arrived. His remarks, although heard, were not addressed at anyone in particular and he received no acknowledgement from any person present. Dr H had some matters to discuss with Mr P.

When Mr P arrived on the ward, a junior doctor Dr L, who had only been on the ward for 5 weeks, took responsibility for the case. He had to get a specialist registrar to oversee his lumbar puncture and the administration of the drug and asked Dr M to assist.

Unfortunately, Dr M had only been on the ward for 2 days and this was his first job as a registrar. He had not received any induction training that would have made it clear to him that he should initially only be shadowing the consultant, and not performing or supervising procedures himself.

Neither of the two doctors had any formal training in giving chemotherapy drugs and both wrongly assumed that the other had checked the drugs and knew the correct route of administration. A nurse handed the bag containing both drugs to the doctors and Dr L correctly injected the cytosine into Mr P's spine in a confident and purposeful manner.

Dr M then read out the name and dose of the vincristine but he did not say how it should be administered. Dr L reported that he asked whether the vincristine should be given spinally and he said that Dr M had indicated that it should be. He said he was surprised by this, but had not felt he could challenge a superior.

Dr M suggested to investigators that he had complete confidence in the system to keep intravenous and intrathecal medications separate, as he understood it to have worked at his previous hospital in Leicester. It was revealed that Leicester and QMC had different procedures in this regard. At Leicester intravenous and intrathecal medications were given on the same day but in different rooms. Dr M said that his understanding of the procedures led him to believe that any drugs present in theatre on that day were to be administered intrathecally.

At this point Dr L claims to have queried the route of administration of the vincristine but that Dr M had indicated to him that he should proceed.

Within minutes the mistake was realized and desperate efforts were made to reverse the procedure, but despite emergency surgery it was too late. Mr P's body became slowly paralysed, his breathing started to fail and his parents agreed to turn off his life support machine.

Comment on case studies 6–8

Although the opening scenarios of these three fatal accidents were somewhat different to each other they all generated an almost identical final scene. An inexperienced junior doctor was handed vincristine to inject when he was carrying out an intrathecal injection.

The last two cases involved changes of plan. All three cases also involved communication failures many of which were related to the changes of plan.

All three cases could have been prevented had there been a good induction course for the junior doctors joining the department covering the dangers associated with chemotherapy drugs, local hospital procedures, limitations on which activities junior doctors could carry out, etc.

Case study 9: medication error—miscalculation of dose

A 2-year-old boy was admitted to hospital on a Saturday afternoon as an emergency. He had a fever, was fretful, and had a petechial rash. An SHO made a diagnosis that he probably had meningococcal meningitis and septicaemia. Arrangements were made for a lumbar puncture and for intravenous antibiotics to start.

The registrar told the SHO to heparinize the child. Almost as soon as the SHO had given the heparin, he realized that he had given far too much. He had miscalculated the dose by one decimal point and had given the child 10 times the amount he should have had. He felt dreadful, but did not know what to do.

He called the registrar and explained what had happened. He came immediately to help and advised that the child be given an injection of protamine sulphate to reverse the effects of the heparin. The next 12 hours were the worst of that SHO's life as he waited to see if the boy recovered from both the heparin overdose and the meningitis. Luckily the boy did survive.

Comment

Always ask someone to check your arithmetic. It is easy to miscalculate the dose of a drug.

Case study 10: medication error—frequency of administration mis-prescribed as 'daily' instead of 'weekly'

Mrs C, a frail 86-year-old lady, was suffering from rheumatoid arthritis. Her rheumatologist, Dr R, started methotrexate.

Dr R explained to Mrs C that she would need to carry on taking methotrexate, but that she could get future prescriptions from her GP. He advised her that she should come to hospital each month for monitoring and blood tests, although this period could lengthen to every 2 or 3 months once she was stable on the medication. In the meantime, the dose of the tablets could change.

When Dr S, an SHO, wrote Mrs C's discharge prescription, it stated 'methotrexate 2.5 mg once daily'. Dr S did not work for Dr R and was merely covering for the ward where Mrs C had been a patient. She was discharged the weekend after her initial FBC result had come back as normal. Dr S had no rheumatology experience, and was unaware that this medication was usually given on a once-weekly basis. He had previously worked on an oncology ward where daily doses of methotrexate had been used. Dr S did not notice that on Mrs C's inpatient drug chart the drug was to be given weekly. The error was not detected by the normal pharmacy checking arrangements in the hospital. Two week's worth of medication was dispensed.

Dr S did not fill in any clinical or follow-up details on Mrs C's discharge summary. This meant that no rheumatological follow-up appointment or monitoring of her FBC and liver function tests were arranged after Mrs C's discharge.

When Mrs C picked up her prescription, she was surprised to see that she needed to take her tablets more often than usual. She did not say anything to the pharmacist as the hospital doctor had told her that the dose might change.

After taking her methotrexate for about 10 days she had suffered continuous nausea and vomiting that had not responded to over-the-counter medicines. Thinking that she had a bug that was going around, she continued to take the methotrexate.

Mrs C eventually saw her GP who noted that she was taking a daily dose of methotrexate, which he thought was unusual. He had also received a copy of her discharge prescription that lacked the usual clinical details. He phoned the rheumatology registrar to find out more. The error was noticed at that point and Mrs C was seen later that day in the rheumatology clinic. She was neutropenic with a white cell count of $2.1 \times 10^9/l$ and thrombocytopenic with a platelet count of $25 \times 10^9/l$.

Fortunately, Mrs C made a full recovery once the methotrexate had been discontinued. Had the error not been spotted by her GP, she almost certainly would have suffered serious harm.

Comment

Prescribing is intrinsically complex and error prone and requires great care.

When prescribing agents with which you are unfamiliar, check in a reputable formulary, such as the BNF that the indications, dose, frequency, and route are correct. If you are unsure, do not be afraid to ask for help.

Discharge prescriptions and summaries are vital communications between secondary and primary care, not just transcriptions of inpatient drug charts. They should be completed in full by a member of the team that cared for the patient. The discharge summary should give the GP all the information needed to manage the patient in the post-discharge period. Details of follow-up arrangements and of the need for monitoring are particularly important. This information should always appear in a discharge summary. Check that any prescription is clear, legible, and unambiguous. Do not prescribe for long periods of time, especially if the patient is new to taking a particular medicine. This way you can check for any dosing or compliance problems.

Make sure that your patient knows why he or she is taking the medication, how many tablets to take, and what to look for in terms of warning signs of potential side-effects.

Case study 11: medication error—wrong drug

Dr C, a consultant anaesthetist, had started work at 7.45 a.m. By the early afternoon he had had no rest breaks or lunch. He had also recently received some distressing family news.

At about 1 p.m. he went to the controlled drugs cabinet to prepare some 'Hepsal' (the anticoagulant drug heparin, at a concentration of 10 International Units per millilitre in 5-ml bottles), to administer to four children who were to be anaesthetised that afternoon.

He looked in the part of the cabinet from which he had collected Hepsal many times before. He said that sometimes he had found the ampoules unboxed. He was unaware that there was also some *Monoparin* (a low molecular weight heparin, at a concentration of 5000 International Units per millilitre in 5-ml bottles) was stored in the cabinet.

Some weeks earlier an oncology patient who had a surgically implanted central line (a *Vas-cath*) had required *Monoparin* to maintain patency of the device. It was recognized that there would be further patients admitted to the department who would require *Monoparin* as part of their treatment regimen and so the remaining ampoules were not returned to the pharmacy.

The anaesthetist reached into the cabinet and inadvertently picked up the ampoules of *Monoparin*. He did not read the labels on the ampoules correctly and he 'saw' what he expected to see rather than perceiving the information that was physically present. He did not find a colleague with whom to carry out a verbal double-checking safety protocol because he was not aware that the Trusts *Medicines Code* required him to undertake one before the administration of medicines to children.

He then undertook the preparation of all the drugs for all four patients in one batch thus creating the potential for the multiple patient adverse event, which then occurred.

During that evening two of the children who had been treated bled more than normally from the site where tissue samples had been taken. The next morning the department was made aware that the two patients had experienced excessive blood loss. When four ampoules of *Monoparin* could not be accounted for during a routine check of the '*Controlled Drugs Cupboard*' it was realized that an adverse event may have taken place.

All four children had received a significant overdose of heparin. As a result, one child underwent an in-depth investigation, a second child had his treatment schedule slightly modified, while the other two required no changes to their regimens. Thankfully, none of the children appear to have suffered any long-term problems as a result of their overdose of heparin. Nevertheless, this represented a serious adverse event.

Case study 12: miscommunication of path lab result

An SHO was coming to the end of his first week in A&E. His shift should have ended an hour before, but the department was busy and his registrar asked if he would see one more patient.

The patient was an 18-year-old man. He was with his parents who were sure that he had taken an overdose. His mother had found an empty bottle of paracetamol that had been full the day before. He had taken overdoses before and was under the care of a psychiatrist. He was adamant he had only taken a couple of tablets for a headache. He said that he had dropped the remaining tablets on the floor and so had thrown them away.

The parents said that they had found the empty bottle 6 hours ago and felt sure that he could not have taken the paracetamol more than 10 hours ago. The SHO explained that a gastric lavage would be of no benefit. He took blood tests to establish paracetamol and salicylate levels. He asked the path lab to phone the A&E department with the results as soon as possible.

A student nurse was at the desk when the lab technician phoned. She wrote down the results in the message book. The salicylate level was negative. Then he gave the paracetamol result. He said 'two', paused and then said 'one three'. The nurse repeated back 'two point one three' and then put down the phone. She wrote '2.13' in the book.

When the SHO appeared at the desk, the nurse read out the results. The SHO checked the graph on the notice board that showed when to treat overdoses. There was also a protocol for managing paracetamol overdoses on the notice board but this had been covered up by another memo.

The graph showed that 2.13 was well below the level at which treatment was required. The SHO thought briefly about checking with the registrar, but she looked busy. Instead he told the student nurse that the patient would need to be admitted overnight so that the psychiatrist could review him the next day.

The SHO went off duty before the formal pathology report came back from the lab. It read 'paracetamol level: 213'.

The mistake was not discovered for 2 days, by which time the patient was starting to experience the symptoms of irreversible liver failure. It was not possible to find a donor liver for transplant and the patient died a week later.

If he had been correctly treated when he arrived at A&E, he would very probably not have died. The SHO was told by his consultant what had happened on Monday when he started his next shift and, while in a state of shock, explained that he had acted on what he thought was the correct result. He admitted that he had not realized that paracetamol results are never reported with a decimal point. Because he had not seen the protocol he had not appreciated that it might have been appropriate to start treatment before the paracetamol result had come back. There was a history, although contradictory, that suggested the patient may not have taken the tablets.

Comment

This patient died because of the *verbal* miscommunication of a numerical value that the receiver thought included a decimal point. Similar *written* miscommunications involving the decimal point have also occurred with fatal results.

In this case a point was added into the numerical value erroneously. More often the error is to omit the point (understanding 5 mg instead of 0.5 mg) or to misplace it in the sequence of numbers (2.25 instead of 22.5).

In high-risk industries misunderstandings relating to the decimal point can have devastating consequences. As a result safety-critical verbal communication protocols in high reliability industries require the use of the three-syllable word 'DAY–SEE–MAL' instead of the single syllable word 'point'.

The three-syllable word 'DAY–SEE–MAL' is much less likely to be missed or misheard than the little word 'point'. The word 'DAY–SEE–MAL' requires some deliberation to enunciate it clearly, signalling to the receiver that this is a safety-critical communication regarding a numerical value that could be misunderstood.

In this case reliability could have been further enhanced if the sender (the technician) had said that the result was abnormally high. The use of an appropriate opening phrase before the actual data value would have been helpful. For example: 'The result is abnormal. The paracetamol level for Lee Brian Jones d.o.b: 1/3/87 is two hundred and thirteen. That is two–one–three, which is very high'.

The nurse should have repeated the above back. She should also have given the technician the chance to confirm that the read back was correct.

If possible always review a written copy (a print-out) of results. Check the correct value, the normal range and units.

In this case the SHO should have been shown during his induction training where safety-critical protocols were located so that he would have easy access to them.

Case study 13: biopsy results for two patients mixed up

Mr O, a consultant urologist carried out a transrectal ultrasound-guided needle biopsy of the prostate of two patients, Mr A and Mr B. Each sample was labelled with the patient's details and was then sent to the pathology laboratory together with a request form.

The biopsies were made into slides for histological examination. The slides for each patient and the request forms were passed to Dr P, an SHO in pathology. Dr P examined the slide from Mr A and noted down her findings. She did the same for Mr B's slide.

An hour later she took the slides to a consultant pathologist, Dr R to check. Dr P and Dr R reviewed the slides together under a double-headed microscope. Dr R advised Dr P that one sample demonstrated prostate cancer and the other benign prostatic hyperplasia. The other sample was benign. Dr P wrote the consultant's findings on the back of each patient's request form.

Later that day, the SHO dictated the findings from each request form on to tape. She attached each tape to the corresponding request form and gave these to the secretary, who put the details into the computer. The computer generated reports for Mr A and Mr B. The SHO and the consultant double-checked that the information in the reports matched the findings on the request form. They did.

The reports were sent to Mr O, the consultant urologist. He told Mr A that his biopsy did not find any cancer and he did not need any treatment. He told Mr B that the biopsy sample showed adenocarcinoma of the prostate and after a discussion about treatment options Mr B underwent a course of radiotherapy.

A year later Mr O saw Mr A again. Despite the benign biopsy from a year ago, Mr A had a serum PSA that was more elevated than it had been a year previously. So Mr O decided to take another needle biopsy. This time the sample showed adenocarcinoma of the prostate.

Dr R, the consultant pathologist, rechecked the slides of the previous biopsy for Mr B. It was correctly labelled with the patient's details and showed obvious adenocarcinoma; however, the details given in the report stated 'benign prostatic hyperplasia'.

Further investigation revealed that Mr A's report stated that adenocarcinoma was present, but the slides showed no evidence of cancer.

It seemed that when the consultant and the SHO had reviewed the slides, the consultant had correctly diagnosed the cancer but the SHO wrote the diagnosis on the back of the wrong patient's request form. The SHO used the incorrect notes to generate the report.

Mr O met each patient to apologise and explain what had happened. All the prostate biopsy slides the SHO had reviewed were rechecked but no more errors were found.

Most medical errors affect a single patient. In this case two patients were harmed by this single slip up. Mr A was told he did not have prostate cancer when he did. One year's delay in treating him could significantly affect his prognosis. Mr B was subjected to an unnecessary course of radiotherapy.

Comments

This case shows how a single mistake can invalidate all other checks and can have much greater consequences than might first appear, in this case affecting two patients. The consultant confirmed that the computer reports matched the request forms but had no way of knowing that the diagnoses on the request forms were wrong. The following lessons were learned from an analysis of this case.

Similar types of sample should be separated in the laboratory booking-in and reporting process.

When juniors present more than one prostate biopsy for review during supervision, they should be placed in separate trays. When a consultant checks a slide, he or she should check that it matches the identity on the request form before passing it to the junior doctor. The consultant should also sign the request form to show that he or she agrees with the junior doctor's diagnosis.

Juniors and consultants should check computer reports against both the patient identification details and the diagnosis on the request form.

Case study 14: penicillin allergy death

Mrs K, a 68-year-old former nurse, had been making a successful recovery from a hysterectomy at a London hospital when she was given an intravenous dose of Augmentin. Within 30 seconds Mrs K had developed marked angioedema of her face, and marked difficulty in breathing. Unfortunately resuscitation attempts failed and she died.

Over a year before she had developed swelling or her face and mouth after being given penicillin but had survived. As a result, the warning 'severe penicillin allergy' was written on the front of her medical notes. In addition, Mrs K had been wearing a bright red wrist-band carrying the words 'penicillin allergy'.

The doctor who had signed the prescription had not seen the warning because the cover of Mrs K's medical notes had been folded back.

One important problem that contributed to this tragedy was that there was no clear label on the outside of the packaging for Augmentin, stating that it was a penicillin-based antibiotic. This was in spite of the fact that documents provided with the drug contained the prominent warning, 'Not to be used in allergy to penicillin or cephalosporin-type antibiotics'.

Case study 15: missing X-ray report

A newly qualified consultant rheumatologist diagnosed a woman as having dermatomyositis. He organized a cancer screen, including a chest X-ray because of the association with malignancy. The hospital was full so the patient was moved to another ward before the round. When he saw her, the X-ray was not available having disappeared between the previous ward and the current one. All of the other tests were as expected and she was discharged.

Two weeks later the consultant saw her in the outpatient clinic. She was responding well to treatment. The blood tests were repeated but the consultant forgot that he had not checked her X-ray. There was nothing in the discharge report to prompt the consultant to follow-up the X-ray. The X-ray department were very likely to have telephoned about abnormal results but the message was not received by the consultant.

It was several months before he noticed the X-ray report was not in the notes and opened the envelope to look at the film. The film showed an obvious tumour, duly identified by the radiologist whose report was still in the envelope. The consultant had to tell the woman that she had cancer and that she would have to be referred to a cancer specialist and that the delay in doing so was his fault.

Comment

This is a depressingly common scenario. If someone presents to A&E then an X-ray may be requested by the A&E staff and the patient is moved on to, say, general medicine—before the X-ray is done.

The request card bears the name of an A&E consultant who quickly forgets the patient. Radiology does not know who is in charge of the patient. Usually, a consultant will look at the X-rays, but non-radiologists often miss incidental small tumours (as indeed do experienced radiologists from time to time).

The paper report is sent days later to A&E (who requested the X-ray, not to the consultant now looking after the patient) by which time the patient could be almost anywhere. An electronic report will be sitting on the system but this may not necessarily be looked at if there are no symptoms or signs referable to the chest, for example, as in this case there were none.

Case study 16: medication not given

In America, a 5-year-old boy had electrodes surgically implanted into his brain to treat his epilepsy. Six hours after the operation, seizures began to rack the boy's entire body and anticonvulsant medication had to be administered immediately. Yet in spite of the fact there were several neurosurgeons, neurologists, and staff from the intensive care unit either at the bedside, on call nearby or at the end of the telephone no one administered the medication. Eventually, a small dose was administered but it was too little too late.

The boy suffered a myocardial infarction and died 2 days later. When investigators asked the doctors and nurses involved how the boy could have died when he was attended by so many skilled professionals, they said that they all assumed that somebody else was responsible for administering the drugs.

The intensive care staff thought that it was the responsibility of the neurosurgeons or the neurologists. The neurosurgeons thought it was the responsibility of the neurologists or the staff from the intensive care unit. The neurologists thought it was the responsibility of the neurosurgeons or the staff from the intensive care unit. Those on the telephone assumed those by the bedside had already given the medication.

Comment

The failure of the teams to carry out an adequate briefing process (about who does what) cost this boy his life.

In many healthcare settings there is no formalized demarcation of work roles. Differing customs and practices develop in different teams and significant hazards arise when staff change teams or different teams work together. The result can be:

- 'Things that ought to be done are left undone' (as in this case), or
- 'Things that ought to be done, are done twice.' (see 3rd case on p. 160)

Case study 17: oesophageal intubation[7]

An anaesthetic registrar, Dr D, lost 'situation awareness' during a procedure to drain a tooth abscess. The patient, Mrs Q, a 39-year-old mother of three died the following morning.

In spite of highly effective procedures developed over many years to prevent oesophageal intubation Dr D made this elementary error. The expert witness at Leeds Coroner's Court, Professor C said that the anaesthetist had 'latched on to the belief' (= adopted the mental model) that he had placed the airway correctly in the trachea. He seems to have maintained this 'belief' for over 3 minutes 'when readings suggested otherwise'.

Professor C said that a consultant anaesthetist, Dr M, who was called to help 'made a serious error when he failed to challenge Dr D's claim the tube was in the right place'. Sadly, Dr D had completely failed to notice the very obvious clue that the patient's stomach was distending. Another doctor said that the patient looked as if she was pregnant.

Comment

Perception is highly influenced by our expectations and we have a tendency to see what we expect to see. Thus we may fail to see things that we are not expecting to see—in this case the distending stomach.

Case study 18: tiredness error

A consultant rheumatologist was tired after a long outpatient clinic but needed to dictate the letters to be sent out to each patient's GP. The last patient that had been seen was a woman with rheumatoid arthritis. She was prescribed sulfasalazine and in the letter to her GP the consultant said that blood monitoring was not required.

A few days later the GP rang the consultant to say that he would usually monitor patients taking sulfasalazine. The consultant immediately realized his mistake. Monitoring is essential because people taking this drug are at risk of serious bone marrow failure, liver damage, and kidney damage. It turned out that the consultant had been thinking of hydroxychloroquine for which haematological and blood monitoring is not required.

The consultant told the GP that he had made a mistake and was deeply apologetic. Fortunately, the patient did not come to any harm.

Comment

It is especially easy to make a mistake when you are tired or are carrying out a familiar routine, in this case dictating a batch of similar letters about patients with similar problems. Luckily in this case there was an alert GP who had the confidence to question a specialist's advice. You might not be so lucky.

Case study 19: inadequate training

Dr J, an SHO, had been working in the paediatric department for 6 weeks. She had had 3 days of induction training. It was departmental policy that registrars should accompany new SHOs to deliveries for the first month.

It was mid-afternoon and the SHO had been called to the labour ward to attend the delivery of a term baby. The mother was fully dilated but her second stage had been delayed. The obstetrician had been concerned about the CTG trace for 10 minutes.

Soon after the SHO arrived a baby boy weighing 3.4 kg was delivered. He was immediately placed on the paediatric resuscitation unit. The SHO dried and wrapped the baby, opened the airway to a neutral position and, concerned that the baby did not cry and appeared generally flat, assessed his heart rate and breathing. As the baby was not breathing she gave five inflation breaths with the bag and mask. His heart rate was approximately 60 bpm and his APGAR score was recorded as 3.

The chest was still not moving so she reassessed the airways and repeated the inflation breaths, this time using a Guedel airway. She started to bag and mask the baby but his heart rate remained low at 70 bpm. She checked the position of the baby and of the Guedel airway, which seemed satisfactory.

As the clock ticked past the 2-minute mark, the SHO estimated that the APGAR score remained at only 3. She would need to intubate the baby if the situation did not improve quickly. She had not performed a paediatric intubation before. Her only experience of intubation was with adults as a medical student on her anaesthetics attachment 3 years before. The model used for practising paediatric intubation was broken and so she had not received any practical training in this technique.

At about 2 minutes and 40 seconds, the SHO asked the midwife for a 3.5-mm endotracheal tube and to call the registrar urgently for help. In the meantime she stopped bagging and masking and opened the laryngoscope. She attempted to pass the laryngoscope through what she thought were the vocal cords but immediately met resistance. She tried again but the tube would not pass.

The midwife came back into the room to say that the registrar was on SCBU dealing with a severely unwell premature baby. He promised to join the SHO as soon as possible, agreed that intubation was needed right away and called the consultant for help. The consultant was in clinic and would take at least 5 minutes to arrive.

The SHO resumed bagging and masking and asked for a smaller 3-mm endotracheal tube. This time it appeared to pass between the vocal cords successfully. The clock showed nearly 4 minutes had elapsed. The SHO inflated the baby's lungs and, listening to the chest, heard faint breathing sounds. She saw his chest rising and falling, but the midwife remarked that the chest inflation seemed poor. The baby's heart rate had increased to 100 bpm.

The consultant arrived a minute or so later and quickly arranged for the baby to be transferred to SCBU. Once the baby was stabilized on a ventilator he decided to reintubate using a larger diameter tube to reduce gas leakage. The baby could not be weaned off the ventilator for 6 days. Cranial ultrasound revealed significant intraventricular haemorrhages and hypoxic ischaemic encephalopathy.

Comment

The phrase 'damned if you do, damned if you don't' comes to mind with this case. It is easy to say that the SHO was not trained to intubate and therefore should not have done it. However, the baby would have been hypoxic until senior help arrived. She had no option but to go ahead and most doctors would have done the same.

The error happened because the system let the SHO down. She was untrained because the training equipment was broken. She was unsupervised because the Trust did not provide adequate senior cover.

We can learn several lessons from this case:

◆ *If SHOs are expected to perform procedures on their own they must be trained.* The Trust should provide such training before the need for it arises. Training equipment should be checked and maintained.

◆ *If policies say that registrars must accompany new SHOs to deliveries, then staffing levels should allow for this.* A dedicated consultant presence for SCBU/NICU, rather than consultant cover from a clinic would prevent such errors.

◆ *All doctors need to be aware of their competency levels and work within them.* In this case the SHO appeared to do her best in the circumstances; however, these circumstances should not have arisen.

There are a few things that SHOs could do to prevent similar errors.

- Consider calling for help early if you need it. In this case the SHO was in a difficult position because both the registrar and the consultant were unavailable, but she needed to get senior help as soon as it became apparent that she could not ventilate the baby with bag and mask.

- Regularly review your resuscitation skills, and request further training if necessary.

- Always check resuscitation equipment before you need to use it.

Case study 20: patient fatality—anaesthetist fell asleep

An 8-year-old boy was admitted to a hospital in Denver, Colorado, for elective surgery on the eardrum. He was anaesthetized and an endotracheal tube and temperature probe was inserted.

The anaesthetist did not listen to the chest after inserting the tube. The temperature probe connector was not compatible with the monitor (the hospital had changed brands the previous day). The anaesthetist asked for another but did not connect it.

Surgery began at 08.20 and carbon dioxide concentrations began to rise after about 30 minutes. The anaesthetist stopped entering CO_2 and pulse on the patient's chart. Nurses observed the anaesthetist nodding in his chair, head bobbing; they did not speak to him because they 'were afraid of a confrontation.' Nor did they draw this to the attention of the surgeon.

At 10.15 the surgeon heard a gurgling sound and realized that the airways tube was disconnected. The problem was called out to the anaesthetist, who roused himself and reconnected the tube. Once again the anaesthetist did not check breathing sounds with his stethoscope.

At 10.30 the patient was breathing so rapidly the surgeon could not operate; he notified the anaesthetist that the respiratory rate was 60 per minute. The anaesthetist did nothing after being alerted.

At 10.45 the monitor, warned of a marked arrhythmia, but the surgeon continued to operate. At 10.59 the anaesthetist asked the surgeon to stop operating. The patient was given a dose of lignocaine, but his condition worsened.

At 11.02 the patient's heart stopped beating. The anaesthetist summoned the emergency cardiac arrest team. The endotracheal tube was removed and found to be 50% obstructed by a mucous plug. A new tube was inserted and the patient was ventilated. The emergency team anaesthetist noticed that the airways heater had caused the breathing circuit's plastic tubing to melt and turned the heater off. The patient's temperature was 42.2 °C. The patient died despite the efforts of the emergency resuscitation team.

Comment

A thankfully rare case of culpable behaviour! Had the theatre nurses been given training in how to 'speak up' this could have allowed them to alert the anaesthetist of problems as they occurred and to have asked for help from the surgeon if the anaesthetist failed to heed their requests.

References

1. http://www.bmj.com/cgi/content/extract/324/7352/1476/6
2. **Dyer C**. Doctors go on trial for manslaughter after removing wrong kidney. *BMJ* 2002; **324**: 1476.
3. **Dyer C**. Doctors cleared of manslaughter. *BMJ* 1999; **318**: 418.
4. Department of Health. *An organization with a memory*. London: Department of Health; 2000.
5. http://www.dh.gov.uk/en/publicationsandstatistics/publications/publications policyandguidance/DH_4010064
6. **Dyer C**. Doctors suspended after injecting wrong drug into spine. *BMJ* 2001; **322:** 257.
7. http://www.gmc-uk.org

Chapter 5

Error management

Error management is the science and practice of controlling or mitigating human error and is a fundamental discipline in high reliability organizations. When applied systematically it is highly successful: the evidence from high reliability organizations is that error management procedures can reduce catastrophic human errors to extremely low levels. It does not generally require expensive or complex technologies. Many of its practices are disarmingly simple.

How accidents happen: the person approach versus the systems approach

In the same way that correctly identifying a disease is necessary before selecting the proper course of treatment, it is important to understand, with an appropriate level of detail, the pathogenesis of adverse events in order to manage effective corrective solutions.

There is a temptation when analysing the cause of error to assume that accidents arise from inadequate medical knowledge or skills or from aberrant mental processes, such as forgetfulness, inattention, laziness, low motivation, or clumsiness. In a limited number of cases this can be true. Bad things do happen to bad people. Sloppy or reckless operators will clearly have more than their fair share of incidents.

However, the overwhelming majority of human error accidents in healthcare, as in other safety-critical industries, involve good people who may be either having an 'off day' or, more frequently, are the unwitting victim of a convincing but deceptive *set of circumstances*, which fate has arranged to entrap them.

One might take solace in the thought that this will not happen to me: 'I will always be careful; I will never screw up'. Comforting though this thought might be, evidence from aviation and other safety-critical industries suggests that even the most meticulous and conscientious operators *will*, from time to time, fall victim to malevolent coincidences that induce serious errors. As we will see later, there is a particular type of error to which the expert is prone—simply because he or she *is* an expert. So, expertise does not guarantee immunity from error.

Many of the world's worst aviation disasters, including the worst of all time, involved highly experienced and well regarded pilots whose competence had, until their last flight, never been questioned.

Allocating blame

News of an avoidable fatal accident often produces a strong emotional response. A common way of dealing with this emotion can be to find someone to blame. The media have found that stirring and exploiting these emotions with 'outrage-generating' language sells more newspapers and boosts TV news ratings. Even highly reputable newspapers and journalists indulge themselves in this form of error analysis.

The belief that such accidents are the result of one or more culpable errors by one or more culpable individuals is known as the 'person approach' to error analysis. The 'rationale' behind this method of error prevention is that if the guilty person can be found and removed from the organization the problem is solved and the error cannot possibly occur again. The others will then be frightened into being more careful. From time to time we have heard doctor and nursing colleagues using this approach to error prevention, with statements such as: 'If I was in charge I'd sack the next nurse who made an error like that on a drug round', or 'We don't pay consultants all that money to make mistakes'.

These glib comments might sound good, but as an approach to preventing error they are absolutely doomed to failure. First, the work force in any healthcare organization would be decimated, quite literally, within a matter of weeks, because *every* healthcare worker commits errors (not infrequently serious ones). Within a year there would be very few doctors and nurses left working in any hospital. If we take the railways as a parallel, many (perhaps all) train drivers will, at some time in their careers pass a signal at danger (a so-called SPAD, 'signal passed at danger'). Fortunately for the travelling public, railway management has embraced the systems approach to dealing with this problem. Rather than sending train drivers who pass signals at danger on gardening leave or firing them, highly effective systems have been developed to prevent or mitigate the effects of SPADs. These systems involve a systems approach to why signals are passed at danger together with human factors training for train drivers.

Of course, the visceral blame approach to error analysis is an understandable, though regrettable, aspect of human psychology. We all like to blame someone when something goes wrong (though we find it difficult to blame ourselves!). However, this approach is also a guarantee that a sustainable way of eliminating subsequent errors will *not* be found.

We know from high reliability organization analyses of accidents that the overwhelming majority of accidents are initiated by faults in the 'system' rather than by lazy, culpable, good for nothing doctors and nurses. The 'systems approach', as used by high reliability organizations, suggests that minimizing these systems failures is the key to preventing accidents.

Error chains

Some years ago the human factors training community developed the term 'error chain' to describe the sequence of events that leads to an accident. This focuses our attention not only on the proximate and final error that led to the accident (usually a front-line worker such as a doctor or nurse), but also on the chain of events that lead up to the hapless operator making that error. The significance of this approach is that it allows the use of the analogy of 'breaking the chain'.

Breaking the chain

The old saying goes 'a chain is only as strong as its weakest link'. Personnel in high reliability organizations are trained to 'break the (error) chain' by targeting its weakest point. Some links of the chain can be considered to be harder to break than others. It makes sense to direct attention to breaking the weakest links of the chain.

As we shall see, 'malevolent coincidences' can be very difficult to mitigate, and as such are the strong links of the chain. For example, it might be hard to entirely eliminate the risk of a wrong patient error if two patients named Margaret Ellen Smith happen to be admitted to a hospital on the same day. The only defence against such an eventuality is a robust and consistent patient identification process.

The weaker (and thus the easier to remedy) links of the error chain are:

- communication failures
- poor checking behaviours
- inadequate or inconsistent procedures
- interruptions
- changes of plan.

High reliability organizations target their efforts at these potential sources of error.

Accident causation

In simple terms, an adverse event scenario starts when 'system failures' combine with or induce errors made by the 'operators' (the term 'operator' refers to personnel who work 'on the front line', such as doctors, nurses, pilots, nuclear power plant control room staff, train drivers, etc.).

In the first part of the error chain, the operator errors are often very minor and may occur over a relatively long period of time and in different locations.

This can make them difficult to detect even with robust error detection procedures.

These errors may be caused or noticed by several different people who do not appreciate their significance or their potential to combine with each other to produce an adverse event. A 'large' error during the early stages of an error chain would usually be noticed and corrected. That such a phenomenon exists has been demonstrated by Professor Marc de Leval at Great Ormond Street Hospital, in the context of paediatric cardiac surgery.[1] Major errors are obvious, easily visible and therefore more easily correctable than minor errors that may remain invisible until a major catastrophe is beyond the point of no return. For this reason the cumulative effect of several minor errors can be as deadly, or even more deadly, as a single major error.

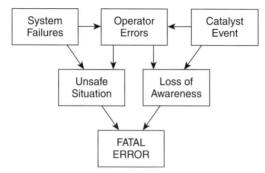

Fig. 5.1 Accident causation model.

Invariably a catalyst, some event outside the control of the system or the operators, supplies the spark to set off the chain reaction (Fig. 5.1). The combination of these elements produces a loss of situation awareness. They may also cause a potentially unsafe situation. Alternatively, the unsafe situation may already exist.

The second stage of the error chain, after the loss of awareness, is generally shorter in duration with operators making a small number of major errors.

Let us apply this analysis to case 1 in Chapter 4 where a doctor erroneously carried out a liver biopsy on the wrong patient, a Mrs T, who in a confused state had got into Mrs K's bed while Mrs K was off the ward (see also Fig. 5.2). Mrs T subsequently died from bleeding due to an uncorrected clotting disorder.

The doctor's error in failing to identify the patient was principally the result of the failure of the hospital system to provide the doctor with training in the 'active identification' of the patient.

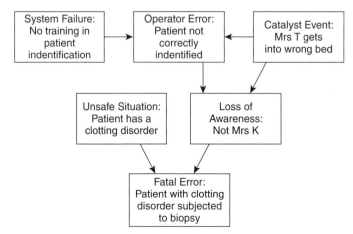

Fig. 5.2 Accident causation model applied to the wrong patient case.

The catalyst event was a confused Mrs T getting into Mrs K's empty bed. The malevolent coincidence of these two events occurring simultaneously caused the doctor to make the wrong mental model about the patient's identity. The fact that the patient appeared to have responded to the wrong name reinforced the wrong mental model.

The unsafe situation was that the patient had a clotting disorder.

Unaware that he had the wrong patient and that that patient had a clotting disorder, the doctor carried out an action that had fatal consequences. On this occasion the doctor believed he was doing the right thing. He had no premonition of the fatal consequences of his action.

System failures

Clinicians generally do not appreciate the part that 'systems failures' play in adverse events. If they are involved in such an event they feel personally guilty and are often prepared to accept more than their fair share of the blame.

It is likely that the doctor in the 'Mrs K's' case (case 1 from Chapter 4) may not have misidentified the patient if he had received formal 'active identification' training. In a high reliability organization this would have been reinforced with regular reminder training and a culture where he saw all of his colleagues consistently checking in the same way. The failure of the hospital to formally mandate 'active identification', train staff in its use and audit compliance is a systems failure. Regular audit of compliance is important, because human beings lapse in their compliance with any process after a time. The 'Forth Road Bridge' analogy is helpful here. Painting the Forth Road Bridge never stops—once it has been completely painted, the process has to start again (so vast is the undertaking that by the time one end of the bridge has been painted, the other end is ready for a fresh coat of paint). Similarly, checking for compliance with safety procedures should never stop and regular training and reminders of procedure form an important part of any safety training process.

Professor James Reason of Manchester University has led academic research into (1) individual human error, and (2) how human errors combine with or are induced by system failures to cause accidents; (3) he has applied his expertise to a number of high-risk areas, including healthcare. He has noted that these system failures, which he calls *latent errors or latent conditions*, are present to varying degrees in all safety-critical industries and share striking similarities.

Systems failures are 'pathogens'—existing situations that may interact with ongoing events to cause operators to make errors or prevent them from detecting them. In other words they can be thought of as accidents 'waiting to happen'. These 'error-inducing' conditions can result from decisions or oversights made at higher levels of management or by the regulatory authorities. Systems failures can include a culture where checks that should be carried out are routinely skipped or where poor performance in others is tolerated.

These threats may remain dormant for many years but, in a great many cases, individuals in parts of the system may be aware of some of them. In healthcare these problems include:

- staff shortages/heavy workloads/lack of time to review working practices
- bed shortages/equipment shortages
- stressful environment/interruptions/frequent changes of plan
- poor protocol design/lack of effective checking practices
- inexperienced personnel working at night
- similar drug packaging/names
- incomplete training and induction/inadequate knowledge or experience
- ergonomic inadequacies with equipment/inadequate maintenance of equipment
- organizational culture that induces or tolerates unsafe practices
- inadequate supervision
- inadequate systems of communication (leading to mishandling of path test results)
- highly mobile working arrangements leading to difficulties in communication
- loss of documentation (e.g. patient records)

- incompatible goals (e.g. conflict between finance and clinical need)
- lack of formal work role assignment (e.g. Who gives an injection?)
- juniors attempting to impress seniors by pretending to be competent in areas where they are not
- culture of infallibility/where errors cannot be discussed
- nurse/doctor cultural divide
- peer tolerance of poor standards (e.g. seeing a colleague carry out an inadequate check of blood transfusion unit but not pointing this out).

Those 'high-risk' industries that have succeeded in reducing accident rates have done so primarily by addressing systems failures rather than by attempting to completely eliminate operator error. The key to solving these problems lies in devising reliable and workable ways of making system failures and latent conditions visible to those who manage and operate the system so that they can be remedied before they combine to cause an accident.

'Catalyst events'

In virtually all error chains there are 'catalyst events'. These include:

- unexpected patient behaviour
- 'malevolent' co-incidence
- changes of plan.

A 'catalyst event' is the spark that ignites the error chain. This is an event that, at the time, is outside the effective control of the operators and thus has a 'disorganizing' effect on the operator's work.

Unexpected patient behaviour and expecting the unexpected

Clinicians know that some patients will not follow instructions, will not keep appointments and may take actions that are not in their best interests. In the majority of cases the clinicians and the system will allow for this. In rare cases the patient's behaviour can be so extraordinary that there are few if any clinicians who would be able to predict what precautions would have to be taken in order to avoid an error from occurring.

On other occasions, the patient's 'error-inducing' behaviour occurs at a time when the system is least able to contain the consequences. Very occasionally, patients will get into the wrong bed! This is very odd behaviour, although perhaps on a ward with a substantial proportion of patients with confusional states or dementia, it may be less unusual.

In the penultimate intrathecal vincristine accident, the catalyst event was the eating, by the victim, of a digestive biscuit. This necessitated the rescheduling of the patient's treatment until later in the day and produced further errors and consequences. This is unexpected behaviour, although it is certainly not unheard of for patients who are supposed to be nil by mouth before a surgical procedure to inadvertently eat or drink something.

Patients sometimes show a surprising lack of understanding of normal preoperative protocol. Just a few weeks ago one of the authors told a 'regular' patient (who was undergoing an operation under exactly the same circumstances as on several previous occasions) that his operation would be done within the next hour, only for the patient to ask 'Can I have a cup of tea then'! It would be easy to assume that this patient should know he was nil by mouth in preparation for a general anaesthetic. There is no accounting for human behaviour! So, in the immortal words of Cardinal Ximinez (played by Michael Palin) of the Spanish Inquisition in Monty Python's Flying Circus, 'expect the unexpected'!

Coincidence (also known as co-occurrence or convergence)

Coincidence is a powerful catalyst in the evolution of error. In the 1989 Boeing 737 crash at Kegworth, there was a fire in the left engine. Unfortunately, the co-pilot misread the cockpit instruments (the layout of the engine instruments was later criticized). He told the captain that the problem was in the right engine. The captain therefore ordered the right engine to be shut down. When this was done, the fire in the left engine *coincidentally* died down for a while. This gave the pilots the illusion that the problem had been correctly handled.

Psychologists studying the loss of awareness associated with such events use the term 'co-occurrence' to describe two or more events that arise simultaneously. On a few tragic occasions a random event may occur at the most inopportune moment and have the effect of confirming a flawed mental model. Equipment failures can also occur at just the wrong moment and cause a distraction.

Changes of plan

Changes of plan are highly productive of error. Reasons for why changes of plan can cause errors include:

- not everyone is informed that the team has now switched to the new plan
- team members sometimes do not have a chance to think through the consequences of the change of plan.

High reliability organizations attempt to organize their operations so that the chance of a change of plan is minimized and formal procedures are developed to handle a change of plan safely.

Anyone working in healthcare will know that changes of plan occur on a very regular basis. At least one reason for this is because the thousands of individual patients that a hospital, for example, has to deal with each year do not always behave in a predictable way. For example, as stated above, patients scheduled for surgery sometimes eat when specifically instructed not to do so. The order of an operating list might therefore change at the last moment to accommodate this.

In healthcare there is little awareness of the potential dangers of changing the plan. However, armed with the knowledge that changes of plan are 'red flags' for error, compensatory mechanisms (such as greater vigilance with pre-operative checking) can reduce the likelihood of an error from occurring.

Human error

So, what is an error?

An error is an unintentional failure in the formulation of a plan by which it is intended to achieve a goal, or an unintentional departure of a sequence of mental or physical activities from the sequence planned, except when such a departure is due to a chance intervention.

> An error is a failure to carry out an intended action successfully—the failure of a planned action to achieve its goal

What is the relative proportion of operator errors to systems errors?

In studies of healthcare adverse events, relative contributions of **operator errors** versus **systems errors** are difficult to determine with certainty since in those studies that categorize types of error, there is wide variation in the relative proportion of operator to systems errors. This is a reflection of the fact that adverse events are very often due to a *combination* of both systems and operator errors (themselves in combination with a catalyst event to start the whole error chain):

- Reason[2] and Runciman et al.[3] have judged that in complex systems in general, a 'systems error' is a contributing factor in accident causation in 90% of accidents (many of these adverse events would also have involved an operator error in combination with the systems error). Conversely, the Quality of Australian Healthcare Study suggested a 'systems error' was a contributing factor in just 16% of accidents.[4] This latter figure is very probably an underestimate of the extent of systems errors in healthcare.

- In the Quality of Australian Healthcare Study, in only 26% of adverse events did the reviewer record the involvement (and type) of operator error that had occurred.

When the types of operator error were identified, these were noted to be: (1) skills based in 26% of cases (so-called slips and lapses); (2) rule based in 27% of cases (e.g. failure to check or failure to follow a protocol); (3) knowledge based in 16% of cases; (4) technical errors in 25% of cases (some error in performing a correct procedure); and (5) violations in 7% of cases (deliberately disregarding a rule or protocol).

Error classification

There are multiple ways of classifying error.

Some systems classify error according to its *outcome*, while others classify error according to its *aetiology*. Other classification systems are hospital or specialty specific, designed by individual hospitals and healthcare organizations as part of their incident-reporting systems, so that staff can classify errors as they occur and report them. Still, other systems are based on the cause or psychological basis for error.

These systems of error classification can be confusing—it is not always obvious to an observer or healthcare worker filing an error report what type of error they are dealing with. Taking a psychological classification system that categorizes errors as errors of action (slips, lapses), errors of knowledge or planning (mistakes), and violations, it can be difficult to determine why an error occurred. Thus an observer may wrongly classify the error, particularly if they are doing a retrospective analysis of a patient's notes. So, giving the wrong dose of intravenous gentamicin may be a **mistake** (e.g. not *knowing* the correct dose in a patient with impaired renal function), a **violation** (deliberately giving a higher dose because of concern that a lower dose may not treat a serious infection adequately), or a **slip** (inadvertently giving a higher dose because you are distracted during the process of drawing up the drug).

Operator errors

Rasmussen and Jensen[5] devised a system of classifying errors—the 'skill–rule–knowledge' system of error classification (also known as the skill–rule–knowledge framework). It is a useful system because it allows us to identify aspects of our own behaviour or that of others that may lead to error.

This framework was based on observations that Rasmussen and Jensen made on the problem-solving behaviour of technicians. They proposed three levels of performance in problem solving:

1 A skill-based level.

2 A rule-based level.

3 A knowledge-based level.

At each level errors can occur. This classification of operator error can be expanded to include two additional types of operator error (not included in Rasmussen and Jensen's original scheme):

4 A violation, where a conscious decision is made to disregard a rule or protocol.

5 A technical error, which is essentially a type of skill-based error.

A 'psychological' classification of errors—one based on how we think and solve problems—allows us to identify aspects of behaviour in healthcare workers that may lead to error.

Identification of error-inducing behaviour allows us to develop more effective ways of preventing error.

'Skill–rule–knowledge' methods of problem solving (after Rasmussen and Jensen)

According to Rasmussen and Jensen's model of three levels of human performance, the cognitive mode in which we operate changes as the task we are performing becomes more familiar—as we become more experienced. In simplistic terms the cognitive mode progresses from the knowledge based through the rule based to the skill-based level.

The task of driving to work provides examples of these three different levels of cognitive processing (see Fig. 5.3 p. 126).

♦ **Errors** are primarily due to human limitations in thinking and remembering—problems with information (e.g. forgetting information, incomplete information).

♦ **Violations** are due to problems of motivation or problems within the work environment.

For example, there may be pressure from hospital management to ensure that no patient is cancelled from an operating list, in order to avoid breaching targets. The surgeon may feel that the only way that the operating list can be completed is by rushing through it and omitting important, but time-consuming safety checks. This could be seen as a *necessary (situational) violation*—necessary to reach the targets—although it is equally easy to argue that the surgeon's prime duty is patient safety and that such a violation is not *necessary*. Giving a drug without checking with another healthcare worker is a common violation, often *situational (borne of necessity)*, because there may not be another member of staff readily available to help with the checking process.

Knowledge-based level of problem solving (or task completion)

Problems are solved or tasks are completed by conscious analysis and stored knowledge (so-called 'deliberative' processing—consciously thinking through a novel task).

- Knowledge-based performance is required when driving along a route you have never driven before. An error in your route is a mistake and it arises because of incorrect knowledge

Rule-based level of problem solving (or task completion)

Problems are solved or tasks are completed by using stored rules which are applied to a specific problem. These rules are based on some previous familiarity with the particular problem at hand.

- Requires recognition of a particular problem followed by the correct application of a rule for managing this problem
- So-called 'if … then' or 'when … then' rules
- When a novice driver negotiates a roundabout he must concentrate intensely to ensure he selects the correct lane in which to approach the roundabout, the correct gear and the correct speed, while signalling appropriately and looking in his mirrors to ensure he doesn't hit another vehicle. He retrieves rules that he has learnt, and applies them to the task:
  - 'If approaching a roundabout to turn right, then look in your mirror'
  - If there is no other vehicle in the right hand lane, then move into the right hand lane'
  - 'When very near the roundabout, change down to third gear' etc.

Skill-based level of problem solving (or task completion)

Problems are solved or tasks are completed by using stored patterns of pre-programmed instructions (learned sequences of skilled actions). The task is familiar and actions to complete the task are taken without conscious thought.

- Attention is consciously directed towards a task only from time to time, particularly at the beginning of the task and at key points requiring decisions during the task. Essentially the task is completed by 'running on autopilot'. Skill-based performance is a very common method of human performance of *routine* tasks.
- Much (if not all) of the cognitive processing during the journey to work of an experienced driver is skills based—he does not need to think of the route, looking in his mirror to negotiate lane changes and roundabouts is automatic, as is selecting the appropriate gear at various parts of the journey

Fig. 5.3 'Skill–rule–knowledge' methods of problem solving. (From Rasmussen J, Jensen A. Mental procedures in real-life tasks: a case study of electronic troubleshooting. *Ergonomics* 1974; **17**: 293–307.)

How experts and novices solve problems

'Experts' tend to rely more on *skill-based* and *rule-based* problem solving—these methods of problem solving are the hallmark of the expert, the hallmark of skilled performance. Experts rely less on knowledge-based (deliberative) processing and as such much of their performance of day-to-day tasks involves operating on autopilot.

Operator errors

Slips and lapses

These are almost invariably due to a failure of attention—due to distraction or preoccupation, typically during an automatic or routine action. Often due to monitoring failures, i.e. failure to check.

♦ *Lapse*: a failure of attention resulting in the *omission* of an intended action (essentially forgetting to do something—an error of memory)

♦ *Slip*: a failure of attention where something is done which is *not intended* (a slip of action = an error of execution)

Technical error

There is no slip, lapse or violation, but there is a failure to successfully carry out the intended action (an incorrect execution of a correct action).

Lapses and slips are characteristic of experts because experts tend to perform many tasks on autopilot (this is part of what defines an expert). Technical errors are characteristic of novices—they diminish in frequency with increasing training, experience and skill. However, even experts will from time to time commit a technical error while carrying out a task.

Mistakes

An inappropriate or incorrect plan that is correctly executed (inadequate plan, actions proceed as intended). Essentially carrying out the wrong procedure (an error of intention; caused by conscious decisions during attempts to solve a problem—so-called problem solving errors).

Rule-based errors

Errors typically involve (1) misidentification of the situation so leading to the use of a rule that is not applicable to the situation (the wrong rule for the situation), or (2) they involve correct identification of the problem, but the incorrect application of the correct rule or failure to apply that correct rule.

The 'rule' used to solve the problem is based on previous experience or training, but for the situation in hand it may be the wrong rule or it may not be applied correctly.

Knowledge-based errors ('deliberative' errors)

Errors arise from incomplete or incorrect knowledge. Knowledge-based errors are characteristic of novices because they rely more on knowledge-based problem solving—and their knowledge base may be inadequate to allow a problem to be solved or a task to be completed. However, experts may also commit such errors. A 'mental model' is developed to attempt to explain what is going wrong, and often 'confirmation bias' comes into play to support this model. There is a tendency to place too much emphasis on evidence that supports this mental model, while ignoring contradictory evidence (which may actually be correct evidence).

Violations

Deliberate deviations from safe operating practices or procedures.

♦ Routine violations (cutting corners whenever an opportunity presents itself).

♦ Optimizing violations (violations to alleviate boredom—essentially for 'kicks').

♦ Necessary (situational) violations (where the rules or procedures are deemed inappropriate for the situation).

Fig. 5.4 A psychological classification of operator errors (based on the 'Skill-rule-knowledge' framework of problem solving—known as the Generic Error Modelling System of error analysis with the addition of technical errors and violations). (From Rasmussen J, Jensen A. Mental procedures in real-life tasks: a case study of electronic troubleshooting. *Ergonomics* 1974; **17**: 293–307.)

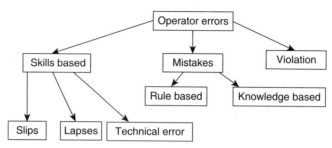

Fig. 5.5 Types of operator error classified according to the 'Skill-rule-knowledge' methods of problem solving (adapted from Rasmussen and Jensen[6]).

'Novices' rely more on knowledge-based problem solving than do experts (though a novice also uses skill-based and rule-based problem solving in task performance). Clearly, because they are novices, their knowledge base is lower than that of experts and there is only so far they can go in solving a problem based on this limited knowledge.

The errors of experts

Rule-based errors become less likely with increasing expertise, because experts develop more comprehensive sets of rules—they have a wider range of stored patterns of problem-solving behaviour based on accumulated experience. They are less likely to make rule-based errors because, based on their accumulated experience, they can recognize a wider repertoire of situations and have a wider and better repertoire of rules to apply to these situations.

Because experts rely proportionately more on skill-based problem solving, skill-based errors—slips and lapses—are characteristic of experts. Skills-based problem solving or task completion uses stored patterns of pre-programmed instructions (learned sequences of skilled actions). The task is familiar and actions to complete the task are taken without conscious thought (essentially tasks are completed on autopilot). Thus, paradoxically, experts tend to be subject to relatively more 'simple' slips or lapses (forgetting to do something) than novices. Expert surgeons are able to complete many steps of a familiar operation on autopilot, possibly preoccupied with something else, but in so doing they may omit an essential safety step (a lapse) such as ensuring that antibiotic or venous thromboembolic disease prophylaxis has been given (the solution is the use of the check-list).

Slips seem to be so simple (on superficial analysis); the fact that they occur is often met with incredulity. We have often heard the statement 'we don't pay doctors all that money to make mistakes', when referring to a seemingly simple lapse or a slip committed by an expert. This demonstrates a fundamental lack of understanding of the nature of expert performance, of expert error and of preventative techniques (see below 'Techniques that *do not* prevent slips and lapses').

- Slips and lapses are failures of attention due to distraction or preoccupation while carrying out an automatic or routine action.
- Slips and lapses are characteristic of experts.

The errors of novices

Because novices rely more on knowledge-based problem solving, they tend to commit relatively more knowledge-based errors than do experts (Virtually all tasks carried out by humans involve both skill-based and rule-based problem solving whether performed by a novice or an expert; however, the skills of the novice are less well developed than those of the expert and the novice has fewer rules to assist performance of a task than does the expert. As a consequence, for both novices and experts, skill- and rule-based errors occur much more frequently than knowledge-based errors; however, the novice commits *proportionately* more knowledge-based errors when compared with skill- and rule-based errors.).

A violation is where an act or decision *knowingly* falls below an expected standard, for example:

- driving at 40 mph in a 30 mph zone
- turning off an alarm on an anaesthetic machine because 'it keeps on going off'.

Techniques that *do not* prevent slips and lapses

- Strict regulation
- Punishment
- Good intentions
- Training*
- The 'incentive' of large salaries*

(*Slips and lapses are characteristic of experts, who are (usually) *highly* trained, well-paid individuals with good intentions.)

None of these 'techniques' prevents such errors because they do not eliminate a fundamental feature of slips and lapses—the fact that they are a form of *human* error. They represent a problem with a fundamental aspect of human cognitive behaviour.

Methods and techniques that *do* prevent slips and lapses

- *Check-lists*: an ordered sequence of rules that must be followed prior to performance of a task.
- *Time outs*: the theatre team (surgeon, anaesthetist, anaesthetic assistant, nurses) discuss a planned procedure in a 'time out' conducted before commencement of the operation.

Three error management opportunities

Fortunately, the vast majority of human errors do not have immediate adverse consequences. Furthermore, most errors are inconsequential.

For other errors there is, in most cases, a period of time between the error being made and its result becoming manifest. Luckily there is usually time to reverse an error. This means that there are three opportunities to 'manage error' (see Fig. 5.6). Let us look at each of these error management opportunities in turn.

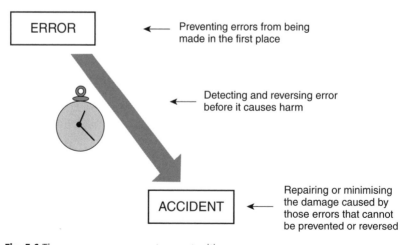

Fig. 5.6 Three error management opportunities.

Preventing error

There are obviously some types of error that *absolutely* must be prevented. These include those errors that are either:

+ irreversible,
+ difficult to detect, or
+ have instantaneous adverse consequences.

In many safety-critical industries there are regular safety courses or safety meetings to remind staff which actions and situations in their department are associated with these critical errors. Very significantly, these courses or meetings frequently reveal that personnel in the same department sometimes have markedly different perceptions of the likelihood of particular errors being made or of their consequences.

There is only limited appreciation in healthcare of the benefits that such courses or meetings can bring. These benefits are not limited to the prevention of error—associated factors contributing to inefficiency can also be addressed. As a result we have seen cases where the same irreversible error has occurred repeatedly without the obvious lesson having being learned.

'Forcing functions'

Forcing functions are elements that reduce the possibility of error by forcing conscious attention to situations where an error could be made. There are:

+ hard forcing functions
+ soft forcing functions.

Hard forcing functions

These are physical features designed into the equipment. One of the earliest known mechanical error prevention systems was introduced to railway signal boxes in 1853. Interlocking levers physically locked track points and signals in a safe position if the signaller erroneously attempted to set the track points in such a way as to cause trains to collide.

The motoring and petrol industries have failed to design a hard forcing function that prevents wrong fuelling. The Automobile Association in the UK estimates that about 150 000 drivers ever year put the wrong fuel in their cars when refuelling—petrol in a diesel engine.[6] The nozzle dimensions are such that petrol can be pumped into a diesel engine car, so there is nothing to prevent the motorist from making this error other than vigilance—which clearly fails 150 000 times a year.

Interestingly, mistakenly filling a petrol engine with diesel is much less common because the standard diesel nozzle at fuel stations is larger than the fuel filler neck on modern petrol cars. As a consequence one has to be very determined and patient to misfuel with diesel as a result. This is a good example of a hard forcing function to prevent diesel fuelling of a petrol engine car. Unfortunately, the lack of a hard forcing function means that the reverse error occurs very frequently.

Medical equipment that is designed to prevent inadvertent drug administration by the wrong route is another hard forcing function. For example, providing only syringes of pre-prepared drugs such as vincristine that will only fit into luer-lock intravenous tubing connections prevents the inadvertent administration of intrathecal vincristine.

Computerized physician order entry systems can include forcing functions that can be programmed to prohibit the ordering of medications until vital patient information such as allergies and weight are entered in the system. It also reduces errors related to handwriting or transcription, can be used to prevent the prescribing of drugs that interact in an unsafe way, allows order entry at point-of-care or off-site, and provides error checking for duplicate or incorrect doses or tests.

Soft forcing functions

These are procedural steps built into work processes. These include the use of pre-operative check-lists, briefings, and verbal double-checking protocols. With a high level of team discipline a high level of compliance can be achieved.

In high reliability organizations personnel are encouraged to have confidence in the effectiveness of checking procedures. As a result compliance is high. In contrast, in healthcare, staff not infrequently have lower expectations of the reliability of checking procedures.

Why not all errors can be prevented

Unfortunately, it is impossible to prevent error completely. Humans are innately fallible because:

- we have limited memory capacity
- stress increases error rates
- fatigue causes increased error rates
- of 'anchoring errors': where a series of recent cases bias the operator toward what seems to be the most likely mental model
- of tunnel vision: ignoring data that disagrees with the assumed mental model
- of left/right confusion and other mental reversals/inversions
- of limited ability to multitask (single channel processing of stimuli).

As a result, the majority of errors may ultimately have to be 'managed' at the second error management level. This is by detecting and reversing error.

Detecting and reversing error

The airline industry has not achieved its success in reducing its accident rates in recent years by breeding a race of infallible pilots. What has changed is that the system now makes it easier to detect and reverse errors. This has been achieved by creating a culture where it is easier to admit, understand, and discuss error.

In this culture everyone accepts the need for standard operating procedures, check-lists, and briefings. They also accept that management is required to carry out audits to ensure that these procedures are applied with sufficient diligence.

The 'detecting-and-reversing-error' strategy includes the following elements:

+ check-lists
+ briefings and announcements
+ standard operating procedures.

In the rare circumstance of these elements failing, the following measures can be used as a final line of defence during an incipient adverse event:

+ 'red flags'—error chain detection system
+ 'speaking up' protocols (e.g. PACE—probe, alert, challenge, emergency)
+ 'alert phrases'—to focus team attention on uncertainties/errors.

Minimizing and repairing the damage

In spite of error prevention and detection measures, not all errors will be intercepted before an accident occurs. When errors cannot be intercepted, procedures have to be in place to minimize the harm caused by the error.

The 1988 Piper Alpha oilrig disaster started with a fire on the drilling deck. Other oilrigs had survived similar fires. Unfortunately, the owners of Piper Alpha had not set up robust procedures to minimize the damage caused by such an event. Massive diesel pumps, which were designed to suck up huge amounts of seawater to dowse the flames, were not switched on. The evacuation plan did not work. The few personnel who survived did so because they disobeyed their safety instructions and jumped over 100 feet into the sea. About an hour after the fire started, it spread to some large high-pressure gas pipes and there was an enormous explosion.

While the 'minimizing-and-repairing-the-damage' error management strategy is obviously the least desirable of the three strategies, training personnel to carry out 'aftermath' activities produces an indirect consequential benefit.

The petrochemical, chemical, and transport industries hold regular exercises to practise the response of the organization and the emergency services to an accident. Such exercises have the important benefit of reminding personnel in high reliability organizations that accidents can happen and this can be an antidote to the complacency that can result from the extremely low accident rate in these organizations. At the end of the disaster exercise the organization can take the opportunity to remind its operators of the importance of adhering to safe operating procedures to prevent an accident of the type that has just been simulated.

Detecting and reversing incipient adverse events in real time: 'Red flags'

High reliability organizations are not immune to disaster and very occasionally the normal error prevention and detection systems do fail. As a result the operator develops a flawed mental model of the operational situation.

> Flaws in mental models can become evident when interactions with the system produce unexpected results.

Analysis of accidents in a range of 'high-risk' industries shows that in many cases some of the operators involved had noticed these unexpected results at a time *before* the situation became irreversible. They had noticed that something was wrong. There were even discussions between team members at the time about these 'symptoms' of the error chain.

In the early 1970s it became mandatory to fit all airliners with a CVR (cockpit voice recorder), which recorded on to a looped tape contained within the black box. In the event of a crash the black box would contain a recording of the last 30 minutes of conversation in the cockpit.

Within a few years the industry had acquired a dozen or so recordings of the events in the cockpit leading up to a crash. The lessons learned from studying these recordings played a major role in preventing recurrences.

Many of these recordings contained strikingly similar types of dialogue. In many cases in the last few minutes before the crash there would be evidence that one member of the cockpit crew had noticed that something was going wrong.

One cockpit gauge would be giving a reading that was inconsistent with the others or with the situation the crew thought they were in. Phrases such as 'look at that difference' or 'that doesn't look right' were uttered.

These 'ambiguities' as they were termed would prompt discussions that indicated confusion. Phrases to the effect of 'I can't understand why this is happening' or 'this doesn't make sense' were recorded. The word 'sure' would often occur as in 'Are you sure?' or 'I'm not sure about this'.

There would also be evidence of unease. The tone of the voices would change, becoming tremulous and phrases such as 'I don't like this' would be blurted out. In one CVR recording the crew talked about how 'scared' they were.

In a few cases every one in the cockpit succumbed to this confusion and unease. More frequently, however, the captain was heard to be denying the unease of the others. Among the final words spoken would be phrases such as 'We're in good shape now' or 'No problem, no problem'.

An error chain can be highly insidious and can impair the ability of its victims to detect it, especially in its advanced stages.

> Victims do not appreciate that they are in an error chain. *All they perceive is a few seemingly unrelated trivial distractions and irritations.*

The term 'red flag' is now used in the aviation industry's human factors training to identify signs and symptoms commonly found in developing error chains.

If pilots hear themselves or their colleagues uttering remarks of a certain tone or if they think certain thoughts they should make a statement, using the term 'red flag', to draw this to the attention of the rest of the crew.

> *Alert phrase:* 'I think we have some red flags here'.

This announcement should then prompt the team to reassess the current situation and resolve the uncertainties.

There are about a dozen different types of 'red flag' or error chain/loss of situation awareness symptoms. In fact several of these 'red flags' are actually the same phenomenon, but as they can be sensed differently they are labelled differently in this list (in order to assist recognition in differing circumstances).

Red flags: the symptoms and signs of evolving error chains

Red flag 1: ambiguities/anomalies/conflicting information or expectations/surprises

The most frequently occurring type of 'red flag' are 'ambiguities'. These are also generally the first 'red flags' to be noticed. In the early stage of an error chain the ambiguities tend to be subtle; later they become progressively more stark.

This category of 'red flag' includes unresolved/unexplained conflicts or contradictions between two sets of information, instrument indications or a difference between what is happening and what was expected to happen.

A clinical red flag would be, for example, when a patient responds unusually to a medication.

These ambiguities may reflect:

- a difference between the operators' incorrect mental model and reality
- a difference between one team member's incorrect mental model and another's more accurate one
- a piece of flawed data and a piece of accurate data
- a difference reflecting a second, changed, plan while someone is persisting with carrying out the first plan.

In case 4 (p. 90) a medical student, while looking at the X-rays noticed the difference in the arterial supply to the two kidneys. She saw the registrar clamping a powerfully pulsating artery and said she thought he was removing the healthy kidney because the X-ray showed a poor blood supply to the diseased kidney. This ambiguity was a 'red flag'.

Phrases and thoughts that indicate this type of red flag might include: 'this arterial flow is much stronger than I was expecting', or 'there is no patient of that name on my list'.

Red flag 2: broken communications/inconclusive discussions

We have all had the experience of observing colleagues who are talking at cross-purposes. You, as a third party can see this, but they do not. This is because they are not really listening to each other. During error chains, communication often breaks down. This can be because:

- People are talking about different things (they may be using pronouns and one person might be using the word 'it' or 'him' to refer to a particular person or medication while the other thinks the pronoun is referring to someone/something else).
- In a fast-moving crisis situation, unforeseen or ambiguous events crop up to interrupt the speaker in mid sentence.
- Owing to the confusion of the situation, the speaker cannot formulate a statement or question that makes sense.
- The speaker dares not contemplate the distasteful implications of the message.

Discussions may take place that keep going round the same points in a 'loop' without reaching any conclusion. There may be a series of unanswered questions. The different mental models of the individual team member can mean that they 'don't know where each other is coming from' and this inhibits effective and timely discussion.

Red flag 3: confusion/loss of awareness/uncertainties

A highly insidious effect of a 'confusion' error chain is the mental 'overload' as the victim tries to make sense out of nonsense. Often there are correct and incorrect data available and the operator attempts to fit both into a mental model. Clearly, this is impossible, but so much cognitive effort is devoted to trying to do so that the obvious dangers of the situation are ignored.

+ 'but I thought you said …'
+ 'are you sure? I wasn't expecting that'
+ 'I can't understand why this is happening'
+ 'this doesn't make sense'
+ 'I haven't got a clue why he's asking for this.'

Red flag 4: missing information/missing steps/incomplete briefing

This red flag is frequently seen in adverse event case studies in healthcare. Errors are much more likely when team members have inadequate information. If it is noticed that one step of a process has been missed, possibly due to distractions, fatigue, or stress, other steps may also have been skipped. Before carrying on, the entire situation should be rechecked. If a procedure continues in the absence of radiology images or notes, for example, any further departures from the expected course may necessitate stopping to re-check any relevant information.

+ 'we only had a verbal report of a CT scan before removing the kidney'
+ 'we couldn't get the X-rays up on the screen'
+ 'the registrar was called to A&E, and had to be replaced by the SHO. The SHO therefore missed the first part of the operation'
+ 'I'm sure I didn't see him check the label on that blood unit'.

Red flag 5: departures from standard procedures/normal practices/'work arounds'/'helping out'

In many error chains someone departs from the standard procedure or their own normal practice. This can occur when someone has to 'work around' an organizational problem such as missing information, test results, medical notes, and X-rays. This might be done in order to 'help someone out'.

Departures from standard procedures and protocols are both a cause and a symptom of loss of situation awareness. In some cases the situation that the team members have created for themselves seems to give them no alternative but to depart from the standard procedure.

In other cases people are observed doing things that are not part of normal practice. In case study 7 (p. 97), one nurse noticed that the doctor was not wearing any gloves when administering the cytotoxic drugs. This was an indication that he was not fully aware of the toxic nature of vincristine.

To save time team members sometimes take shortcuts in check-lists or procedures. They may even make up their own unapproved procedures. They obviously feel they can control any resulting difficulties and restore the situation to the standard whenever they wish. Unfortunately, the effects of an apparently minor 'deliberate' error can combine with the effects of other errors, possibly made by other parties, of which they are not aware.

Just like chemical reactions where two innocuous elements combine to form an explosive compound, two or more departures from the standard protocols can have tragic results.

- ◆ 'normally we have two surgeons and one scrub nurse'
- ◆ 'I didn't see him actually check the notes'
- ◆ 'let's go ahead without the X-rays'
- ◆ 'rules are for the guidance of the wise, and for the strict adherence of fools!'

Red flag 6: fixation/preoccupation

An acute 'mismanaged-crisis' error chain can trigger the stress response. This causes the subject to focus on those stimuli that he feels are relevant to solve the crisis. Other team members may notice one team member's fixation on one aspect of a situation while ignoring the bigger picture. It is vital that this fixation is drawn to the attention of the team.

Case 17 (p. 109) seems to be a case of stress-induced fixation or tunnel vision, 'We're going to do this case no matter what'.

Red flag 7: changes of plan

A number of error chains involve a change of plan (case studies 4, 5, 7, and 8, see pp. 90-98).

This might be a change of plan forced on the team by external circumstances that then initiates the error chain. Alternatively during a stressful error chain situation, the team may decide to change a plan that does not seem to be working. There may be insufficient time to consider all of the consequences of the new plan, which may turn out to have a worse outcome than the original plan.

- 'okay that doesn't seem to be working, let's try this'
- 'let's do the second patient first'
- 'this is a case of out of the frying pan and into the fire'.

Red flag 8: time distortion/event runaway

Research by Dr Anthony Chaston and Dr Alan Kingstone of the University of Alberta considered the effect of cognitive effort on the perception of time. They found that the harder the task, the faster time seems to go by. This is a common experience of surgeons who, during the course of an operation, may look at the clock on the theatre wall only to see that a whole hour has gone by, virtually unnoticed. The Elaine Bromiley case as well as case 17 (see p. 108) are examples of this.

Alternatively, under very high levels of stress, for example, in life-threatening situations, cognitive activity speeds up, giving the impression that reality has gone into slow motion. Survivors of traumatic incidents often report that an event that actually took a few seconds to occur had seemed to last several minutes. It might be possible that in these circumstances a clinician may erroneously feel that a normal patient response to a medication is too slow, causing him to unnecessarily administer a second injection.

In the second part of an error chain the hapless victims make big errors. These produce startling results and sometimes the victims respond with what turns out to be another big error. More startling results appear and the pace of events speeds up. There is insufficient time to assess each new troubling event before another succeeds it.

- 'the blood pressure is still dropping'
- 'Oh ****, it's all happening too fast'
- 'We haven't got time for that'
- 'Wow, look—we've been here two hours—I'd have sworn it was just an hour'
- 'how long have we been going now?'

Red flag 9: unease/fear

The unsettling and stressful nature of the situation may give rise to a strong sense of unease, anxiety, or even fear. Autonomic symptoms may occur such as a dry mouth and hair standing up on the back of the neck. A shiver may run down the spine. The stomach feels empty, the heart races, breathing becomes deeper.

Clinicians are trained to respond to cyanosis in a patient: they should be taught to react to the sight of a colleague looking anxious. These physiological 'red flags' occur inside the body of the clinician.

+ 'the staff nurse sounds nervous'
+ 'my SHO is sweating and seems to want to interrupt'
+ 'I don't like what we've got here'.

Red flag 10: denial/stress/inaction

The refusal to accept the situation can have two causes:

+ One innate reaction to a sudden high level of stress is to 'flee'. A surgeon may not feel able to leave the operating theatre so he may 'flee' from reality by denying it.
+ A stubborn team leader who does not accept the implied criticism of his management by the subordinate's unease or confusion.

There are two possible causes of the inaction evident in the last stages of an error chain:

+ The sudden onset of exceptionally high stress produces the 'freeze' reaction.
+ Subjects are so confused they cannot decide on which course of action to take.
  + 'It will be alright, I've done this before'
  + 'No problem, no problem'
  + 'It's going to be okay'

Red flag 11: juniors cut short

The team leader may interrupt dissenting input from subordinates.

+ 'I know what I'm doing, now back off'
+ 'When I want your advice I'll ask for it'.

Red flag 12: alarm bells—in your mind or real warnings from the equipment

In many adverse incidents in 'high-risk' industries, warning systems were activated in time to prevent disaster and were ignored. In the case of the Chernobyl accident and the 1972 air disaster at Staines, near Heathrow, the operators actually turned off the warning system. Obviously, the warnings did not fit into the mental model of the operator and were ignored.

Alternatively, the warnings were perceived as false. This is more likely when the warning system has given false warnings in the past. A warning system that gives a high level of false warnings represents a serious system failure.

Red flags: caveats

- This section should not be taken to mean that you should not depart from standard procedures/clinical guidelines or change the plan. Clearly, this might be the best course of action in many cases. However, it would be wise to be even more alert to the possibility of error when this happens.
- Many error chains will exhibit no identifiable red flags.
- Some red flags may be evident only after the situation becomes irrecoverable (e.g. in case 3 the evidence in the bisected kidney).
- Events that appear to be red flags may occur innocently (e.g. in stressful A&E procedures).

Speaking up protocols

In the Elaine Bromiley case (see Preface) and case studies 4, 5, 7, and 20 (from Chapter 4, see pp. 90, 93, 97, 112) at least one member of the team recognized that something was going wrong or that the team leader seemed to be unaware of an important adverse development.

> Significantly, this recognition occurred at a time when it was still possible to reverse the errors.

In the Elaine Bromiley case and case 4 a team member did speak up but their input was ignored. In the other cases the team members remained silent.

The failure of junior team members to speak up effectively has been a factor in a number of serious accidents in many safety-critical situations in other industries or organizations. These include:

- *The loss in 1893 of the Royal Navy battleship HMS Victoria:* several officers queried the admiral about the clearance between two vessels in advance of his proposed manoeuvre—the two ships subsequently collided and sank. Many lives were lost.
- *The 1977 Tenerife air disaster:* the flight engineer asked the captain if the other aircraft was clear of the runway. His input was brushed aside. Both died with hundreds of others on board.
- *The 1986 Chernobyl accident:* a technician suggested abandoning the power test when it was realized that the reactor was not properly programmed. The world's worst nuclear disaster followed.
- *The 1986 loss of the Space Shuttle Challenger:* a designer voiced and then withdrew his concerns about the integrity of rubber seals in the solid booster rockets. The leak of hot gas from the rubber seals led to the Challenger exploding in mid-air shortly after take off.

> ◆ *The 1988 explosion of the Piper Alpha oilrig:* a technician on an adjacent oilrig was unable to persuade his supervisor to shut off the gas flow through pipes beneath Piper Alpha when there was already a fire on board. The oil rig and 167 lives were lost in the subsequent fire.

These accidents were the worst ever in their particular industries or organizations. As a result of these admittedly rare but highly costly accidents, some high reliability organizations decided to consider whether it would be wise to provide their staff with a 'speaking up' protocol.

Some airlines have adopted a protocol designed by an American Airlines pilot Captain Robert Besco. Other airlines have developed other protocols.

This is a four-step process. Each step in the sequence provides a way to reduce the danger and to increase the probability of an uneventful resolution. Practised intervention strategies can defuse the potential for hostility, which can erupt when the team leader does not acknowledge he is making a mistake.

This intervention strategy is known as PACE.

PROBE, ALERT, CHALLENGE, EMERGENCY

Level 1: probing

The concerned team member should always bear in mind the very likely possibility that *he* has made a mistake in his own mental modelling of the situation. Thus his question should be an attempt to find out why the others seem to have a different mental model to him. Has he missed a part of the briefing? He should ask an appropriate open question (one not requiring a yes/no answer).

If the team leader cannot answer this question satisfactorily there are grounds for moving on to the next step.

Note: In certain situations the confusion produced by the error chain may be so great that the concerned team members may not easily be able to formulate a sensible probing question. In these cases he should proceed directly to level 2. For example, it may not be possible for him to quickly decide which of two anomalies or ambiguities represent evidence of a problem. The existence of confusion in itself may represent grounds for stopping to reassess.

Level 2: alerting

If level 1 does not produce a satisfactory response, the team member should alert the team or team leader to the potential danger that he thinks the present course of action might bring. In this case the concerned team member should clearly say that he is not happy with the situation.

Level 3: challenging

If the team leader continues on the course of action, the concerned team member should adopt a very assertive tone and state that in his view the present situation is unsafe. He should challenge the team leader to explain his actions or change of plan.

Level 4: emergency

It is the duty of any team member to take control of a situation or halt a procedure when it seems that there is a definite danger. Effectively, the team member is saying there is an emergency and 'I am not going to let it happen'.

Note:

If you are a junior member of the team and you feel unable to address your concerns to the team leader directly you should talk to a colleague who can review the reasons behind your concerns and then speak to the team leader. So, for example, if a junior doctor feels uneasy about speaking up to his consultant, he could discreetly approach a more senior junior colleague (a registrar, for example), explain his concerns, and ask the registrar to speak up on his behalf.

Alert phrases

Some airlines have adopted the alert phrases given in bold in the text box below to support the PACE protocol. These phrases appear in their official operational procedures manuals.

- Level 1: probe
  - There is no phrase connected with level 1, the concerned team member should ask an appropriate question (a question relevant to the situation).
- Level 2: alert
  - **'I am not happy, …'**
- Level 3: challenge
  - **'You must listen, …'**
- Level 4: emergency
  - **'I am taking over, …'**

Example of a healthcare application of PACE (probe, alert, challenge, emergency) alert phrases

Level 1: probe 'Mr Jones, would you mind explaining why the CT scan report says the tumour is in the left kidney, but you've made an incision on the right side?' (This may be enough to alert Mr Jones, the surgeon, to the fact that he is operating on the wrong side).

Level 2: alert 'Mr Jones, I am not happy. The CT report says the tumour is in the left kidney. I think you're operating on the wrong side.'

Level 3: challenge 'Mr Jones, you must listen. You're taking out the wrong kidney.'

In this situation many junior surgeons would very probably feel unable to actually step in a take over the operation. An appeal to the anaesthetist and other members of the theatre team might be a better approach to take: 'Dr Smith (the anaesthetist), please would you check the CT report and confirm to us that the tumour is in the *left* kidney.' A sensible anaesthetist will do so!

Error management using accident and incident data

In the early part of the twentieth century the Cleveland Railway Company ran a network of trams in that city in Ohio. In 1926 the company decided to start keeping accurate and detailed records of accidents and incidents.[7] No doubt employees grumbled at the seeming pointlessness of the required paperwork. In 1930 the company started to process the resulting data and produced a quite surprising finding.

It seemed that tram drivers based at one of their depots, Woodhill, were responsible for more than twice as many accidents and incidents per person as the average for the company. Worse still, the data showed that the rate of accidents and incidents was increasing at Woodhill while the rate was falling at every other depot on their network. The managers of the railway had been completely unaware of this situation.

Clearly, the management had to go up to Woodhill and see what was going on.

It turned out that there was no single cause of this high incident rate. There were four main problems.

First, the Woodhill depot had a very large proportion of drivers in their first year of service. It had not been realized before the data were processed that new drivers had an accident rate three times greater than the most experienced drivers. The second problem was the failure of some drivers to recognize hazards on the roads. A third problem was the casual or awkward 'attitudes' of a small number of the drivers. Finally, a small number of drivers had poor vision.

Additional training was provided to the new drivers. A selection process for new recruits was created in which they were judged on their ability to recognize hazards on the road. The awkward squad were given 'counselling'. An optician helped to resolve the eyesight problems. More reliable eye tests were carried out on recruitment and regular check-ups were scheduled for all drivers.

These measures substantially reduced accidents and incidents at Woodhill the following year. This is believed to have been the first occasion in history when accident and incident data had been used to improve safety.

Furthermore, the exercise yielded an unexpected bonus. It was also noted that there had been a significant reduction in the electrical power used by the Woodhill drivers. It seems that the initiative had not only improved safety but it had made the operation more efficient as well.

High reliability organizations accord a high priority to gathering and processing accident and incident data and this informs the refinement of their procedures and training. It is important to note that the data itself does not always provide the reasons for the problems but helps to enable safety managers to ask the right questions.

In order to improve safety an organization must gather accident and incident data. Eventually a large database can be created, which then can be 'data mined' to look for trends not otherwise recognized. This can reveal unsuspected patterns in the locations, timings, or circumstances of adverse events.

Gathering accident and incident data

There are four principal sources of accident, incident, and error data.

1 Formal adverse event/accident reports.

2 Voluntary incident reports:
   - anonymous
   - signed by the operator involved.

3 Mandatory incident reports—signed by the operator involved.

4 'Black box' monitoring systems.

Formal adverse event/accident reports

Accident reports attract more attention than reports of non-damaging 'near misses'. The organization's accountants have to sign cheques to pay for repairs and compensation after an accident. This seems to make managers somewhat more willing to fund safety programmes.

The carefully structured analysis of accident case studies on training courses is a central element in the safety culture of high reliability organizations. Frequently, accident reports reveal how operators actually behave on a day-to-day basis and how procedures are really carried out. This often varies markedly from the required standards. Previously, managers and operators would deny poor compliance but an accident report is difficult to dispute.

Voluntary incident reports

In 1931, Herbert Heinrich published his book *Industrial Accident Prevention*. Heinrich worked for the Hartford Insurance Company and he visited factories to investigate claims for losses following industrial accidents. His extensive and well organized studies showed that for every one major industrial accident there were 29 'minor-injury accidents' and 300 'near miss' events/ 'no-injury' accidents.[7]

While one might argue about the definition of 'minor-injury accidents' and 'near misses', it is now accepted by safety experts that in all 'safety-critical' industries a major accident is usually preceded by a number of 'near misses'. It also likely that a similar situation exists in healthcare. It is important, therefore, that the organization learns from its 'near misses'.

In June 1972, Britain's worst ever air disaster occurred when a lever in the cockpit of a Trident airliner was moved prematurely. This error, if not reversed within a few seconds, would literally cause the aircraft to fall out of the sky. The airlines' management had been completely unaware that this danger existed. After the accident several pilots came forward to admit that they had made the same error, had managed to reverse it in time and had kept quiet about it. This accident prompted efforts to set up an anonymous incident reporting system in aviation.

In response to the vast costs of catastrophic events, NASA, the aviation, the nuclear power, petrochemical processing, and steel production industries have set up non-punitive, protected, voluntary incident reporting systems for reporting near misses and adverse events. These organizations have assisted each other and shared their experiences in setting up and running such systems. For example NASA helps to run a critical incident reporting system for healthcare professionals in the USA.

These reporting systems produce large amounts of essential information unobtainable by other means and have evolved over the past three decades. The organizations now believe that incident reporting systems benefit their organizations far more than they cost. Not only do they reduce waste but they can actually increase production by removing operational inefficiencies as well as error-inducing situations.

The same underlying circumstances invariably precede both catastrophic events and near misses. 'Near misses' represent a valuable learning opportunity— 'free lessons'—available at no cost in terms of injury or damage.

In the past there were often powerful disincentives for operators to report 'near miss' events. These inhibitions were created by the organizational culture and a fear of punishment.

All NHS Trusts now operate critical incident reporting systems. As a clinician it is your duty to report errors and error-inducing situations that you encounter in your work. In the long term a culture of incident reporting will bring great benefits to healthcare.

Mandatory incident reports

Aviation has decided to make the reporting of certain types of events mandatory. While operators are rarely punished for the errors that result in the incident, failure to report an incident that requires a mandatory report is viewed seriously.

'Black box' automated monitoring systems

These are systems that 'detect' errors without the operator having to make a report. This has been called the 'spy in the cab' (or cockpit). A growing number of high reliability organizations use automated monitoring systems to detect not only dangerous situations but hazardous actions by employees. Most large airlines now download data from the black box flight recorders in their aircraft once a week. The data are run through a computer to detect any 'events' where a pilot has placed his aircraft in a hazardous position. Under an agreement with the pilot's union, the airline is not permitted to take disciplinary action as a result of events detected by this method.

In the five or so years that this 'operational flight data monitoring' has been in use the number of 'events' detected has declined steadily. A pilot is now aware that his chief pilot will be able to see exactly how he is flying the aircraft. As a result the incidence of macho behaviours, such as continuing a steep and fast approach, have reduced markedly. This system encourages pilots to be more cautious in their flying. The results of the annual review of operational flight data monitoring data are fed back to pilots on their annual human factors courses.

Why clinicians might be reluctant to report their critical incidents

Critical incident reporting systems in healthcare are in their infancy. Clinicians may be reluctant to report their errors or error-inducing situations they encounter. The reasons for this may include:

- ◆ lack of awareness of the need to report, what to report, and why;
- ◆ lack of understanding of how to report;
- ◆ staff feel they are too busy to make a report;
- ◆ too much paper work involved in reporting;
- ◆ the patient recovers from the adverse event and the urgency goes out of the situation;
- ◆ fear of the 'point-scoring' by colleagues, retribution by line management, disciplinary action, or litigation;

- an assumption that someone else will make the report;
- no evidence of timely feedback and/or corrective action being taken resulting from making a report.

> **Do take the time to make a report; it will help make healthcare safer and ease your work in future years.**

References

1 de Leval M, Carthy J, Wright DJ, *et al.* Human factors and cardiac surgery: a multicenter study. *J Thorac Cardiovasc Surg* 2000; **119**: 661–72.

2 **Reason J.** Safety in the operating theatre Part 2: human error and organizational failure. *Curr Anaesth Crit Care* 1995; **6**: 121–6.

3 **Runciman WB, Webb RK, Lee R, Holland R.** System failure: an analysis of 2000 incident reports. *Anaesth Intensive Care* 1993; **21**: 684–95.

4 **McL Wilson R, Runciman WB, Gibberd RW, *et al.*** The Quality of Australian Healthcare Study. Medical Journal of Australia 1995; **163**: 458–71.

5 **Rasmussen J, Jensen A.** Mental procedures in real-life tasks: a case study of electronic troubleshooting. *Ergonomics* 1974; **17**: 293–307.

6 http://www.theaa.com/motoring_advice/fuels-and-environment/misfuelling/html

7 **Heinrich HW.** *Industrial accident prevention.* New York: McGraw-Hill Book Company Inc.; 1931.

Further reading

Chang A, Schyve PM, Croteau RJ, O'Leary DS, Loeb JM. The JCAHO patient safety event taxonomy: a standardized terminology and classification schema for near misses and adverse events. *Int J Qual Health Care* 2005; **17**: 95–105.

Gaba DM. Anaesthesiology as a model for patient safety in health care. *Br Med J* 2000; **320**: 785–8.

Hollnagel E. *Cognitive reliability and error analysis.* Oxford: Elsevier; 1998.

Leape LL. Error in medicine. *JAMA* 1994; **272**: 1851–7.

de Leval M, Carthy J, Wright DJ, *et al.* Human factors and cardiac surgery: a multicenter study. *J Thorac Cardiovasc Surg* 2000; **119**: 661–72.

Runciman WB. Lessons from the Australian Patient Safety Foundation: setting up a national patient safety surveillance system—Is this the right model? *Qual Saf Health Care* 2002; **11**: 246–51.

Runciman WB, Helps SC, Sexton EJ, Malpass A. A classification for incidents and accidents in the health-care system. *J Qual Clin Pract* 1998; **18**: 199–211.

Chapter 6

Communication failure

Shortly after 1 p.m. on Friday 18 September 1997 a HST ('High Speed Train') travelling from Swansea to Paddington was entering the outer western suburbs of London. It was still travelling at its cruising speed of 125 mph, although in about 7 minutes it would have to start decelerating for its arrival at the terminus.

Unfortunately at this point, as it passed through Hayes station, its driver failed to notice a double yellow signal that was warning of an unexpected obstruction about five miles ahead. The driver should have immediately started to slow his train. Two minutes later, while passing Southall station, the driver failed to notice a second yellow signal warning him that the next signal would be a red STOP signal.

One minute later the driver was horrified to see the red signal ahead and, some distance beyond it, a long heavy goods train crossing his track. With the train still travelling at 125 mph there was now insufficient time to stop. The impact speed of the HST with the hopper wagons of the goods train was estimated to have been between 80 and 90 mph.

Seven passengers died in the Southall rail accident.

The proximate and principal cause of the accident was clearly the inattention of the driver. However, a secondary factor was revealed. The train's AWS (Automatic Warning System) was faulty. The AWS sounds a horn in the driver's cab when the train approaches amber or red signals.

Before the train had left Swansea there had been two telephone calls to the train company's maintenance headquarters about the fault. Unfortunately, both of these telephone communications had been misunderstood or mishandled. If these messages had been handled correctly, another locomotive with a functioning AWS could have been provided for the train.

Thus two communication failures, 3 hours or so before the fatal impact, had played a part in this disaster.

Reviewing a series of other recent railway accidents and 'near misses', railway safety officials noticed that communication failures play a part in a significant proportion of adverse events. In most cases the communication failure was not the most obvious factor in the accident, but it often played a part in setting up the conditions for a fatal error to be made.

At that time the railway industry had recently started to keep tape recordings of safety-critical telephone and radio conversations between train drivers, signallers, and track maintenance engineers. Auditing these communications, safety officials noted that many of these conversations were of poor quality.

In many cases the diction was unclear. Ambiguous terminology was used. Contrary to existing communication protocols, in about three-quarters of cases vital instructions and messages were not repeated back to the message sender to confirm understanding.

It was clear that sloppy communication behaviours created significant potential for catastrophic misunderstandings. As a result, the railway industry started a programme of Safety Critical Communication skills training for all drivers, signallers, and track maintenance engineers.

Other safety-critical industries have also had cause to adopt formalized protocols to enhance the effectiveness of communications relating to safety-critical matters.

The prevalence of communication failures in adverse events in healthcare

Any organization that depends on the performance of multiple human beings is prone to errors of communication by virtue of the fact that those individuals must communicate in order to perform their job. Therefore, in primary care there are relatively fewer opportunities for errors of communication, where much of a doctor's job is carried out by that individual doctor working in (relative) isolation from other healthcare workers. Conversely in hospital practice, particularly where a patient spends several days or weeks in hospital, the process of care inevitably requires communication between many individuals and teams of individuals, e.g. nurses, doctors (house officers, registrars, consultants), radiologists and radiographers, anaesthetists, and administrative staff such as secretaries and ward clerks.

Many safety-critical industries take the time to compare and study the root causes of *groups* of similar adverse events. One seminal observation results from this research, which is that in spite of the differences in the causes of these events, there is in many cases some type of *communication failure* during the hours and minutes that preceded the accident. A similar finding applies to many adverse events in healthcare.

Sometimes a communication failure directly causes an error with immediate and tragic consequences:

During the resuscitation of a baby in a US hospital, the doctor called for calcium chloride. The nurse thought she heard him say potassium chloride. She administered this substance to the baby with fatal results. It cost the hospital $2 million to settle the consequent legal action. If the nurse had repeated back what she thought she heard doctor say, the accident might not have happened.

In other cases a communication failure, several hours (or even days) before the fatal error, was merely one of a series of different events that set up the conditions that later caused the fatal error. The parties involved may have even been aware that there were uncertainties resulting from the communication failure but did not feel that it was worth following these up.

Parker and Coiera[1] reported in 2000 that in a 'retrospective review of 16,000 in-hospital deaths [in Australia], communication errors were found to be the leading cause'.

Communication errors were 'twice as frequent as errors due to inadequate clinical skill.'

In the USA, an analysis[2] of 2455 serious healthcare adverse events revealed that communication failures were one of the primary root causes in 70% of cases. Reflecting the seriousness of these occurrences, approximately 75% of these patients died. Eighty per cent of wrong site surgery cases were found to have involved a communication failure.

Lingard et al.[3] reported the results of an observational study of 42 surgical procedures in a Toronto hospital. During the 90 hours of observation there were a total of 421 verbal communications between members of the surgical team. Each communication was assessed with respect to 'occasion' (appropriate timing), 'content' (completeness and accuracy), 'purpose' (whether the message achieved its objective, or could have done), and 'audience' (whether the person addressed could have answered or whether key personnel were present). One hundred and twenty-nine communications (30.6%) observed in the operating theatre 'failed' in one or more of these ways. Lingard et al. noted that 'a third of these resulted in effects which jeopardised patient safety'. They found that 'critical information was often transferred in an ad hoc, reactive manner and tension levels were frequently high'.

In the USA, Barenfanger *et al.*[4] studied the rate of communication errors in outgoing telephone calls from diagnostic laboratories. These calls communicated the results of urgent pathology tests (e.g. biochemistry, microbiology) to requesting clinicians and other healthcare workers. The receiving healthcare workers were asked by the lab staff: 'To ensure you have the right information, please repeat the name, test and result I just gave you.'

When the recipient of the message was asked to repeat the test result that had just been relayed to them, in 29 of 882 (3.5%) cases they gave an incorrect reply. In 10 of the 29 cases the healthcare worker repeated the wrong patient's name, and in nine of the 29 cases the recipient repeated an incorrect result. In many cases the doctor was going to initiate treatment based on these misunderstood results. Imagine if incorrect information was received about a patient's serum potassium level. A wrongly communicated serum potassium level could have disastrous consequences. Imagine if the receiving doctor mistakenly thought the potassium was low, and decided to give intravenous potassium to correct this, when in fact the potassium was above the normal range to start with!

Thus we have four studies,[1-4] each looking at different aspects of communication failures in healthcare and using different approaches and methodologies. All of these have found substantial or at least very significant rates of communication error. This situation clearly demands urgent remedy.

It is important to note that communication failures are not distinct from other aspects of healthcare organization and teamwork. They reflect general problems in the way healthcare is organized and the behaviours and attitudes of personnel in the system.

In healthcare there is also a general lack of awareness of the extent of communication failures between clinicians and the very significant adverse effect that these communication failures have on outcomes. There have been no systematic attempts to educate clinicians about the damaging consequences of communication failures.

A doctor's years of training and experience can bring great benefit to his patients. He may correctly diagnose the patient's condition and select the most effective treatment. Unfortunately, if a message relating to the patient's treatment is misunderstood by a colleague, the patient may be harmed. In such a case all that training and experience may have been wasted.

One might conclude from this that it might be beneficial to delete 1 day of training from the clinical syllabus and substitute it with a good 1-day course aimed at improving communications between clinicians. Few medical schools at present provide any clinician-to-clinician communications skills training focused on the typical types of communication failure.

This chapter is intended to draw together some ideas from different domains to help clinicians understand the nature of communication error and give some advice to enhance effective communication.

Communication failure categories

When embarking on a new area of science it is often useful to begin with a taxonomy. A large, seemingly unwieldy, problem can be broken down into 'bite-sized' chunks.

Some elements of a situation might be easy to understand and thus easy to deal with. Other elements may be more complex and require deeper consideration. However, if the easier issues are dealt with first, there will be more resources to apply to the less tractable problems.

Communication failures within and between teams in safety-critical domains can be divided into the following categories:

1 Absent messages (failure to communicate at all).

2 Messages with content problems or inappropriate 'tone' (e.g. missing or incomplete data).

3 Message addressing problems (e.g. speaking to the wrong person).

4 Selecting the wrong communication medium (e.g. telling a colleague something rather than writing it down in the patient's notes).

5 Communicating at an inappropriate time (e.g. distracting a colleague engaged in a highly safety-critical work with a less urgent communication).

6 System failures (e.g. inadequate communication channels, lack of communication skills training).

Communication failure category 1: absent messages/failure to communicate

Absent messages are the failure to originate, transmit, or pass on a required or appropriate message at the appropriate time. (Note: If this failure to communicate is due to the failure of the organization to provide reliable media/communication channels, this would be a system failure—category 6, see below.)

Two major safety-critical industries—the aviation industry[5] and the railways system[6]—have found that 'failure to communicate' is the most common type of communication failure. As a study into communication failures on the railways in Great Britain reported,[6] 'it appears that simply not communicating when one should is a widespread and serious problem.'

There are currently no data on the incidence of 'failure to communicate' as one of the types of communication failures that occur in healthcare. The authors of this book believe that the situation in healthcare in this regard may not be greatly different from other safety-critical industries.

The railway study[6] analysed 391 safety incidents on the railways caused by communication failure and found 'the greatest number of errors were due to a failure to communicate at all'. About one-third of these failures to communicate were found to have been the result of a deliberate decision not to communicate. Another third were the result of not realizing that a communication should have been initiated. Other failures to communicate were the result of distractions by other tasks or forgetfulness.

When comparing healthcare with the railways we may speculate that the putatively steeper hierarchy in healthcare (where juniors may be reluctant to speak up) might produce an even greater rate of *deciding* not to communicate.

However, it might not only be junior doctors who fail to communicate. Senior doctors have also failed to communicate when this would reveal that they have made a mistake or do not know something they might be expected to know.

Case studies

The following case studies from Chapter 4 involved an instance of 'failure to communicate':

+ *Case study 4 (wrong-sided nephrectomy).* The consultant failed to say he had not actually examined the patient's notes even though there was doubt as to the correct side for the nephrectomy.

+ *Case study 5 (wrong site surgery).* The SHO did not speak to the consultant about his fears that a wrong site surgery error might be made.

+ *Case study 7 (intrathecal vincristine).* The nurses failed to point out to Dr G that the consultant always wore gloves when administering vincristine. Had they done so the doctor's attention might have been drawn to the extreme danger associated with this drug ('If it's too dangerous to touch with my hands, what will happen if I inject it intrathecally?').

+ *Case study 20 (anaesthetic problem).* The theatre nurses observed the anaesthetist apparently asleep but they did not draw this to the attention of the surgeon.

Other cases of 'failure to communicate':

- In one case, a doctor inserted a needle into a patient's left side to drain a pleural effusion.[7] At this point the patient said 'I thought it was supposed to be done on the other side'. The doctor then carried out the procedure on her right lung, and in the process created a bilateral pneumothorax. Shortly after this the patient suffered a myocardial infarction. The doctor failed to communicate his error to anyone. Emergency staff who subsequently had to manage the case were, therefore, unaware of the bilateral pneumothorax and as a result failed to recognize the left pneumothorax.

- In another case, an 84-year-old woman underwent urgent surgery for a hiatus hernia. She developed respiratory difficulties for which she was treated with a minitracheotomy. She had a calcified trachea, so a sharper, stouter minitracheotomy tube was inserted. During the night, the physiotherapist was unable to find a suction catheter of the correct diameter to fit down the minitracheotomy tube.

  She telephoned the consultant who had inserted it. He advised her to check if one was available in the ITU. He assumed that she would telephone back if a suitable suction tube was not found. Unfortunately, no suction tube was found but she did not telephone back. The patient died of sputum retention during the night.

An absent communication also played a major part in the world's worst offshore petroleum industry disaster, the Piper Alpha oil-rig explosion. On the afternoon of 6 July 1988 an overhaul of pump 'A', one of the two gas pumps on the oil-rig was planned to start. The maintenance team had only managed to remove the pump's safety valve before their shift ended at 6 p.m. The maintenance engineer returned to the control room to brief the supervisor on how the work was progressing and to hand in a worksheet that showed the status of the pump.

When he entered the control room he found the supervisor deep in conversation with other engineers. After waiting for a while it seemed to him that these conversations would not end quickly. He was reluctant to appear rude and interrupt them so he chose not to communicate. Instead he left the worksheet in a prominent place on the supervisor's desk. It is likely that other paperwork was subsequently placed on top of the worksheet.

At 10 p.m., 4 hours after the 'absent communication', gas pump 'B' failed. Control room operators decided to turn on gas pump 'A'. It was essential to maintain gas pressure in the pipelines and to get either one of the two gas pumps working again as soon as possible. Engineers were aware that maintenance work had been scheduled for pump 'A' and searched the control room for worksheets relating to the pump. The relevant worksheet could not be found. A quick examination of the pump appeared to suggest that it was complete. Unfortunately, the absence of the safety valve was not easy to see from the place at which the engineers were standing.

As soon as pump 'A' was started, inflammable gas escaped from the pipe where the safety valve should have been. This was ignited by an electrical spark and there was an explosion.

The maintenance engineer's failure to communicate, borne of 'politeness', led to the loss of 167 lives and the total destruction of a $1 billion oil-rig.

Solutions to 'failure to communicate'

- Awareness of the potential consequences of failure to communicate.
- Speaking up protocols (e.g. PACE see Chapter 5).
- Pre-operative briefings that confirm what information is already known and what information is needed by which team members.

Communication failure category 2: messages with content problems or inappropriate tone

These are cases where a communication is passed to the correct person at the appropriate time but the communication fails. This might be due to:

- insufficient data (missing elements)
- incorrect data
- excess data (leaving the message receiver to work out what are the relevant data)
- inappropriate emphasis, tone, or body language during data transmission.

The railway study into communication failures[6] found that the majority of this type of communication failures were the result of one party making incorrect assumptions about the other party's intentions, situation, problems, or knowledge.

In healthcare we also see evidence of flawed assumptions causing similar communication errors. In consequence the sender omits data that he believes the receiver already knows or does not need to know. Wrong assumptions about the information that the other party needs can lead to the wrong information being given.

The use of non-specific terminology—particularly the use of pronouns (he, she, it)—falls into this category. A clinician will have a particular patient, medication, or treatment plan in mind when he communicates with a colleague. Unfortunately, if the message does not give the name of patient, medication, or treatment plan and if the message receiver has a different mental model there is the possibility of a misunderstanding.

As stated above, one particular hazard lies in the use of pronouns. These seemingly innocuous little words take the place of nouns and names, but (without wishing to sound melodramatic) their use has led to many deaths (see the Norwich–Yarmouth rail disaster example)! Thus we do not have to keep saying 'John Smith' whenever we talk about John Smith. We refer to him as 'he' or 'him'. However, if we have also been speaking about Joe Brown, there is a possibility that the words 'he' or 'him' could be misunderstood to refer to the wrong person. Other pronouns include 'it', 'this', 'that', 'she', 'her', and 'there'. The inappropriate use of pronouns can result in medications, objects, patients, and places being confused.

Non-routine messages

Another problem that falls into this category is where a non-routine message is not handled appropriately. Examples include messages relating to:

- emergencies
- abnormal, unusual situations
- changes of plan (e.g. changes to operating lists or personnel rostered to carry out a particular activity).

In these situations the communication error might occur if the receiver does not appreciate that the message requires special attention. The Frenchay Hospital Study, Bristol, 1995[8] observed and analysed the communication behaviour of eight physicians (ranging in grade from junior house officer to consultant) and two nurses while they carried out their duties in a general medicine department. The doctors who received pages were observed to have to guess the urgency of incoming 'page' (messages). It seemed that they would ignore some pages and assume that a second page from the same ward meant that the message might be urgent.

Category 2 communication failures can have fatal consequences as is shown in the following case studies.

Case studies

Five of the 20 adverse event case studies in Chapter 4 involve an instance of this type of communication failure during their error chains.

- *Case study 2*: the tone of the anaesthetist's voice inadvertently suggested urgency when he asked the nurse to get the blood unit. There was actually no particular urgency as there was no significant blood loss at that time.

However, the rush may have contributed to her failing to check the blood unit correctly.

- *Case study 4:* the medical student did not give (and was not given the chance to explain) her reasons behind her question: 'Aren't you taking out the wrong kidney?'.
- *Case study 6:* the consultant's secretary's message to Dr P about the patient's appointment time on the following day was incomplete. There was also a misunderstanding about exactly what parts of the procedure Dr S would be supervising.
- *Case study 7:* there were misunderstandings in the face-to-face discussion at 10.45 and also in the telephone call immediately before the fatal error.
- *Case study 12:* miscommunication of a path lab result.

An ambiguous message can be misunderstood if an apparent gesture or a form of body language seems to suggest the wrong interpretation.

Communication failure: error of content (specifically the use of a pronoun leading to a disaster)

An example of this type of communication failure occurred on the platform of Norwich station on the evening of 10 September 1873.[9] Every evening at 9 p.m. an express train from London stopped briefly at Norwich before continuing to Yarmouth. At that time the railway between Norwich and Yarmouth was a single-track line. When the express reached Yarmouth, a Royal Mail train would leave Yarmouth for Norwich to return down the single-track line.

That night the express from London was running late. The station inspector suggested to the stationmaster at Norwich to reverse the sequence and allow the Royal Mail train to use the single-track line first. It would be given permission to set out from Yarmouth on time. The stationmaster objected to this because it would delay the express further while it waited for the Royal Mail train to reach Norwich. The inspector correctly pointed out that the railway company would incur a penalty under the contract with the Post Office for delaying the Royal Mail train. He told the stationmaster, 'There is an official company order allowing us to detain the express until 9.35 p.m.'. The Royal Mail train would have been able to reach Norwich by then. According to the company order, the inspector was right and the Royal Mail train should go first.

To this the stationmaster made an ambiguous reply. With a shrug and a tone of impatient dismissal he said 'All right, ... we'll soon get *her* off'. The inspector evidently believed from his body language that the stationmaster had conceded his point and that the word 'her' must refer to the Royal Mail train. The inspector sent a telegram to Yarmouth authorising the Royal Mail train to set out. He was unaware that the stationmaster had already sent a telegram to Yarmouth advising them that the express would go first.

When the express arrived at Norwich the stationmaster handed the driver a copy of his telegram as his authority to enter the single-track section. The express soon set off towards Yarmouth. Hearing the sounds of the express starting off, the inspector dashed out of the office to tell the stationmaster that he had already authorised the other train to set out as well.

The inspector rushed back to the telegraph office and a desperate two-word message was sent to the other end of the line: 'STOP MAIL'

In an instant the numbing reply was received: 'MAIL LEFT'

While the two stricken men stood helplessly on the platform at Norwich station reeling at their ghastly and irreversible error, a tragedy was about to happen in the blackness beyond the station lights.

At 9.30 p.m. the two trains met in a thunderous head-on collision at the Yare Bridge. Twenty-five people died and 73 were injured!—All because of a misunderstood pronoun and an ambiguous piece of body language.

Solutions to 'incomplete data' etc

- 'Read back'.
- Use of opening phrases/alert phrases.
- Avoiding the use of pronouns.
- Studying adverse event case studies, which resulted from incomplete data being passed.
- Pre-operative briefings that confirm what information is already known and what information is needed by which team members.

Communication failure category 3: message addressing problems (e.g. speaking to the wrong person)

It seems that this type of communication failure occurs somewhat less frequently than the first two types. However, it may be proportionately more likely to have lethal consequences than the first two categories.

One reason for the high 'lethality' of such communication errors is that in this type of case there is often very little time to reverse the error.

Instructions from air traffic controllers that are passed to the pilots of the wrong aeroplanes or signallers who mistakenly address the drivers of the wrong trains can create an extremely hazardous situation very quickly.

When a doctor treats the wrong patient (other than a patient in a coma or under anaesthesia) he/she will almost certainly be speaking to him/her, thus presenting an example of this type of communication failure.

There are several variations on message addressing problems:

> 1 'A' intends to address 'B' but does not realize he is really speaking to 'C'.
>
> 2 'B' believes he is receiving a message from 'A' but it is really a message from 'C'.
>
> 3 'A' addresses 'B' but 'C' overhears and carries out the instruction as well.
>
> 4 'A' does not address his remark to any named individual and the people who hear it all assume the message is intended for someone else.

Failing to address a message properly can have serious consequences as can be seen in case studies.

Case studies

Two of the 20 adverse event case studies in Chapter 4 involve 'message addressing' failures.

- *Case study 1:* the SHO spoke to (and carried out the procedure on) the wrong patient with fatal consequences.
- *Case study 8:* the consultant addressed his request to be told when the patient arrived towards several members of the ward staff. He received no acknowledgement from any one of them, with everyone assuming that somebody else would carry out his request.

Other message addressing failures include:

- During resuscitation of a patient with severe burns the doctor gave a verbal order for intravenous morphine but did not address the instruction to any one person. One nurse administered the morphine. A moment later a second nurse, unaware that the injection had already been given, gave a second injection. The patient's breathing started to slow down. Fortunately, the error was detected and quickly reversed.
- One day in 1873 at Menheniot station in Cornwall on the Great Western Railway two trains were waiting to depart.[9] One was heading east, the other west. When a message came through from the next signal box to the west

that the last westbound train was clear of the track section, the signalman was able to give permission to the westbound train to proceed. He leaned out of the signal box window and called out to the guard: 'Okay, Dick off you go!' Tragically, by coincidence, the guard of the eastbound train was also named Dick. The eastbound train also started off and could not be stopped. Five minutes later it was involved in a head on collision with another train. The driver and fireman of the eastbound train were killed.

Solutions to addressing problems (see below for detailed discussion)

- Identify yourself and who you are talking to.
- 'Active identification' of patients (asking the *patient* to confirm who they are, their date of birth and address).

Communication failure category 4: selecting the wrong communication medium (e.g. sending an email rather than speaking directly to someone on the phone)

Initially, one thinks of a communication failure as a misunderstanding between two individuals during a face-to-face or telephone conversation. In fact the scope of the types of communication that can play a part in adverse events is very much greater. The table below categorizes the different types of communications media available to clinicians.

Methods of communication between healthcare workers

- Verbal
  - face to face
  - telephone conversation
- Pager
- Written
  - entries made in hospital notes
  - letters to other healthcare workers
- Handovers between shifts
- Electronic hospital records
- Email
- Internet (e.g. lab results)
- Fax

Selecting a medium that is inappropriate to the nature of the message can contribute to error. Sometimes clinicians use verbal communication when a written note would be more appropriate. Conversely, they may rely on a written note when the circumstances necessitate their immediately verbalizing the idea.

In some situations the 'belt and braces' approach, the use of two independent media might provide adequate reliability for important safety-critical messages.

In the Frenchay Hospital communications behaviours study,[8] clinicians were observed to have a preference for the use of immediate (synchronous) communications such as face-to-face conversations or telephone calls for messages in situations where non-synchronous media, such as written notes, might have been equally effective. There was a tendency to seek information from colleagues rather than looking it up in documentation. The authors of the study speculated that this preference might have been because immediate (synchronous) communications provide evidence that the message has been received by the receiver. It was also suggested that the reliance of the subjects on conversation to resolve information needs is in response to poor documentation. Another hypothesis is that as clinical problems are often poorly defined, reassurance and clarification can be obtained through conversation. Thus, medical staff may opportunistically interrupt each other because face-to-face discussion is highly valued but difficult to organize in advance, and any opportunity to communicate is avidly seized.

This behaviour was observed to be highly interruptive of the receiver's work. Interruptions can cause distraction that lead to errors.

The use of the fax machine to send urgent communications is a good example of a form of communication where errors can occur. Accident and emergency department staff and general practitioners frequently send urgent communications by fax, the assumption being that the fax will always get through (that there will definitely be someone at the other end of the communication who knows how to act on the urgent situation appropriately). Sometimes the fax is preceded by verbal communication from the 'sender' to the 'receiver' of the communication, the fax in this situation merely serving to communicate the patient's details (name, address, etc.) and acting as a formal referral, for example. Such communications tend to be important—hence the reason for sending a fax rather than simply sending a letter by post—and they usually require urgent action of some sort or other. Sometimes, however, the sender of the fax simply sends the fax without any verbal communication. The message sender hopes that the receiver will receive the communication and act upon it. The potential for error is obvious. The message may fail to get through because:

- the fax number may be wrong
- the fax machine may be out of paper so delaying receipt of the message
- the staff who 'attend' the fax machine may be away (sending urgent faxes on a Friday afternoon is a recipe for a delayed communication!)
- the doctor for whom the fax is concerned (the doctor who must 'action' the information contained therein) may be on leave for the next 2 weeks, the person who picks up the fax may not appreciate its significance and it may sit in an in-tray until his return from leave.

As a consequence of any of these problems getting in the way of the fax getting through, a safety-critical communication may end up never being communicated or at the very least an urgent communication may take weeks to be acted upon! We have seen examples of all of the above communications failures.

Using the wrong medium for a safety-critical communication can have serious consequences. In case study 5, the SHO should have written a warning in the patient's notes rather than relying on a verbal communication the following day.

Communication failure category 5: communicating at an inappropriate time

In the Frenchay Hospital communications behaviours study,[8] clinicians were observed to interrupt each other frequently even when the 'interruptee' was obviously busy attending to their work.

In interviews after the observation the subjects rarely considered the effect that their communication could have on the other party's work. Their actions could thus be characterized as habitual and selfish in that they valued completion of their own tasks over their colleagues' tasks.

In the Toronto study[3] of communications within surgical teams, the most frequently observed type of communication failure was also what they termed 'occasion failure'. This is where subjects were observed to communicate at inappropriate times:

- Communicating about a less important matter when the message receiver is busy with safety-critical work or otherwise distracted.
- Communicating while there are temporary adverse environmental factors (e.g. loud background noise from equipment).
- Communicating too early.

The nurses and the anaesthetist were observed to discuss how the patient should be positioned for surgery before the surgeon arrived in theatre.

Sometimes these discussions led to decisions that later had to be reversed when the surgeon arrived and the patient had to be repositioned. On other occasions there were conversations between nurses and surgeons about anaesthetic issues before the anaesthetist arrived. Not surprisingly, these conversations failed to achieve their purpose.

- Communicating too late (more frequent than communicating too early).

Many of the communications were 'reactive', relating to situations that ought to have been resolved before surgery commenced. On one occasion, 1 hour into the procedure, the surgeon was observed to ask whether antibiotics had been administered. It seemed they had not. Prophylactic antibiotics are optimally given within 30 minutes of the first incision. This is a common problem.

Communication failure category 6: system failures

The healthcare system appears to suffer enormous inefficiencies because of poor communication infrastructure and practices. One estimate[10] suggested that the US health system could save $30 billion per annum with improved telecommunications.

In the Frenchay study,[8] clinicians were observed to waste considerable amounts of time attempting to communicate on the telephone. Many of these problems could be resolved relatively easily by a small number of very simple measures.

For example, a *series* of calls was often required to book an investigation. One senior medical registrar was observed to make eight phone calls (three failed to connect) and one page over a 54-minute period to arrange one CT scan. Thus for the best part of an hour his medical skills and knowledge were unavailable to other patients. Another subject, a nurse, made two pages (both unanswered) to medical staff and two phone calls to a clinic over 12 minutes in an unsuccessful attempt to organize an endoscopy. Such sequences usually involved the caller following a trail of telephone numbers, reflecting a lack of thought on many sides.

Some subjects were unsure about which individual to contact to organize an investigation, e.g. 'who do I call to arrange a venogram?'. One specialist nurse who dealt exclusively with elderly patients was repeatedly paged in error to see patients outside her area of responsibility. The hospital's phone directory was partly structured around roles, but gave no indication of what tasks or responsibilities were associated with a role. It would be very simple to issue a more 'user-friendly' hospital phone book.

Learning from (communication) errors and communicating the lessons learnt

Many high reliability organizations provide staff with regular training courses and publications that examine communication error case studies. From these, staff become aware of the typical and recurring communication failure types. Thus when they compose a safety-critical message they tend consider how that message might be misunderstood.

Whose fault: message sender or receiver?

Most professional people believe that they are good communicators. Doctors clearly have to be highly articulate in order to gain entry to medical school and to progress through medical training and graduate.

There is a strong tendency for both parties to a failed communication to blame the other. Message senders often believe that it was the receiver's fault for not paying attention. The message receiver on the other hand might complain that the message he received was incomplete.

Who is right, who is at fault—the message sender or message receiver?

The authors believe that a study into communication failures on the railways in Great Britain[6] provides an answer that also applies to healthcare. This study found that in 58% of cases of communication error, the person who initiated the communication, or should have done, was solely responsible for the error.

In a further 21% of cases both parties were at fault. This might have been because the message was confusing or incomplete but the receiver failed to ask for clarification or point out that he had not understood it.

> If we add these two percentages, we see that the message sender was either fully or partly responsible for the communication error in 79% of cases.

It is very likely that the overwhelming majority of communication errors in healthcare are also the fault of the message sender.

The lesson to learn from this is that message senders should take care when composing a message.

In healthcare we frequently hear message senders make statements along the lines of 'I told the SHO to check the serum calcium and he didn't', which is said in such a tone as to chastize the SHO for not listening! It is conceivable, and in fact often likely, that the message sender did not speak clearly (poor diction), or did not specify which patient's serum calcium should be measured, or did not specify which junior doctor should actually complete the request for the blood to be taken for the serum calcium to be measured. It is possible that he made the request when the receiver was busy recording the details of the ward round in the notes or when the receiver was being interrupted in some other way, such as by a pager going off. Perhaps the SHO simply did not hear the request for the serum calcium to be checked. The SHO is only human after all!

The message sender may want to rant and rave about the failure of the SHO to check the serum calcium, but he could save himself, the patient, and the SHO a lot of trouble simply by confirming that the SHO received and understood the request for the serum calcium to be checked. At the end of the ward round or at the consultation with a given patient, the message sender could simply ask the message receiver to repeat back what has been requested, e.g. 'Let me just double check that you got down everything I asked for—what blood tests are you going to do …?'.

If communications' senders took the time to structure the message adequately and took responsibility to ensure that the receiver understood the message then misunderstandings would be less likely to occur.

Safety-critical communications (SCC) protocols

At 5.04 p.m. on Sunday 27 March 1977 there was a terrible misunderstanding over the air traffic radio between the pilots of a Boeing 747 and the control tower at Tenerife airport.

The pilots had passed an ambiguous communication to the control tower about taking off. The controller in the tower had thought that they were saying that they were in position on the runway and were waiting for permission to take off. The controller replied 'OK, … stand by for take-off'.

Unfortunately, radio interference had masked the words 'stand by' and the cockpit voice recorder shows that the pilots heard the words 'OK, … (unintelligible) for take-off'. The controller's voice seemed to have a positive tone. The captain took this to be a clearance to take off.

Less than a minute after this communication failure 583 people had burned to death in a huge fireball. The aircraft had collided at 140 mph with another fully loaded Boeing 747 that was hidden behind a bank of fog that had just rolled across the runway.

As a result of this catastrophe the protocols for giving and receiving take-off clearances were completely changed. Henceforth pilots would report that they were 'ready for departure'. They were prohibited from saying that they were 'ready for take-off'. The control tower would then reply either 'cleared for take-off' or 'hold position'. The pilot would then 'read back' 'the controller's words. Pilots and controllers were prohibited from using the words 'take-off' in any other circumstance.

Thus pilots could no longer ask, for example, 'which runway is in use for take-off?' or 'which route will I follow after take-off'. The word 'departure' was to be used instead of 'take-off' except for the actual positive take-off clearance and its read back.

Following these changes, there has never been a repeat of this disaster.

Many safety-critical industries have suffered immensely costly accidents that were the result of communication failures between personnel. In order to prevent further disasters, high reliability organizations have adopted a range of standardized procedures for safety-critical communications (SCC).

These procedures can be highly effective:

> The railways study[6] reports that they believe they have had *not one single* adverse event resulting from a communication failure where both parties to the communication correctly followed the industry's SCC protocols.

Definition

An SCC is any communication that could produce the risk of harm if it is:

- misunderstood
- not sent or sent at an inappropriate time
- misaddressed/misdirected or acted upon by the wrong person.

Safety-critical communication protocols: elements

- 'Taking the lead'
- 'Read back', paraphrased 'read back'.
- Identifying the parties to a communication
- Clear diction and use of 'standard English'
- Opening phrases/alert phrases
- Standard message structures/sequences of data
- NATO phonetic alphabet
- Avoiding non-pertinent communication/communicating at an inappropriate time/non-standard terminology
- Awareness of communication failure scenarios

'Taking the lead'

One might take the view that successful communication should depend equally on both parties. Provided you 'do your bit' and the other party 'does their bit', everything should be OK. Thus, it seems that once you have delivered what you think is an appropriate message it might seem that your responsibility is fulfilled. While this attitude might seem to be appropriate, trainers of SCC procedures believe that a much more vigorous attitude toward SCC is necessary.

Their advice is that you should take 'lead responsibility' to ensure that each SCC to which you are a party is successful. You must assume that the communication will fail unless you take positive measures to ensure that it does not.

'Lead responsibility' must also apply if you are the receiver of a message. If you receive an incomplete or confusing SCC from the other party you should take responsibility to ensure you extract the correct meaning from the sender.

> In other words, the person 'taking the lead' not only has to follow all the relevant rules and procedures themselves but has to make sure that the other person does too.

The advice given in the text box below is taken from a Network Rail publication.[11] It reflects the similarities between communications issues in different safety-critical industries such that it is reproduced below without a single amendment, needing no changes to be relevant to healthcare:

> 'Taking the lead' involves a number of responsibilities:
> - Identifying who you are and who you are talking to so you know it's the right person
> - Listening to the other party and the information they are giving
> - Questioning the other party, when appropriate, to ensure they have all the information available in order to decide on the correct course of action.
> - Challenging the poor communications style of others and prompting the other party to use the communication protocols
> - Correcting any mistakes when the other party is repeating the message back
> - Calming the other party down if agitated or angry
> - Repeating back the message/information provided and prompt the other party to repeat back any message/information he/she has provided
> - Concluding the conversation appropriately by summarizing and/or ensuring the other party is clear about what is required

We not infrequently see entries in hospital notes such as 'Dr Jones has not answered his page' or 'Dr Smith has failed to return my call' or 'Unable to contact Mr Jones'. There is almost a 'tone' of censure, as if to imply 'Well, I've done my job and the fact that he hasn't answered (hasn't received my message) isn't my fault'. At other times there is an implication that the message receiver has wilfully refused to answer the page. One almost feels like writing a suggestion after such comments such as 'must try harder to ensure his communication gets through'! In this era of modern communications, where many people have a mobile phone or pager, there is really very little excuse for not trying again if a communication does not get through the first time. And if the message doesn't get through to a specific member of a team, try another team member until your request *is* satisfied.

If you are sending a safety-critical message, your job does *not* stop once you have sent the message. Your job stops only once you have confirmed that the proposed message receiver has actually *received and understood the message*. If you have made every effort to contact the proposed message receiver and have failed, contact someone else in the team to ensure your safety-critical message does get through.

'Read back'/paraphrased 'read back'

> THE SINGLE MOST IMPORTANT TOOL TO PREVENT
> MISCOMMUNICATIONS IS 'READ BACK'

'Read back' is the practice of repeating back a verbal 'safety-critical' message to its sender and receiving confirmation from the sender that the 'read back' is correct. It is thus a three-step process:

1 the passing of the message from sender to receiver
2 the repeating back of the message by the receiver to the sender
3 the sender stating that the 'read back' is correct.

Clearly, this three-step process is only appropriate for safety-critical communications where a misunderstanding could result in harm. Its use for other messages would be irksome. Read back has two benefits:

◆ **receipt** of the message can be confirmed, and
◆ **understanding** can (usually) be confirmed.

We use 'read back' in everyday life when we use a telephone banking service to transfer money from one account to another. The bank repeats back to you the sum of money and names of the accounts involved. It is a very common behaviour to repeat back a phone number you have taken down in order to ensure you have the correct number. When we order a home delivery pizza, the details are repeated back. One might ask if it is appropriate for a pepperoni pizza should it not also be appropriate for 'read back' to be used for SCC in healthcare—Is it worth checking that the junior doctor who you asked to administer potassium chloride to a patient has heard the dose you want given correctly?

Receipt confirmation

It can be dangerous to assume that because you have sent a message to someone, that they will receive that message. Clinicians sometimes email a request to someone and assume that their request will be carried out. The 'emailed' person may, for example, be on leave and might have forgotten to switch on their 'out of office' auto reply.

This is a classic example of the message sender assuming that their only responsibility is transmission of the message and that once the 'send' button has been clicked, their responsibility stops there—that the message has definitely been received. The safe approach is for the message sender to assume the message has not been received/understood/acted upon until the message sender has received positive confirmation to the contrary.

Understanding confirmation

In straightforward situations the receiver will understand the message. If the message has implications these might need to be more explicitly stated.

Use of 'read back' in healthcare

We have already noted Barenfanger *et al.*'s study[4] found that 3.5% of telephone calls communicating the results of urgent pathology tests were misunderstood. The process of requiring the recipient to 'read back' the result corrected *all* these errors.

In the USA, the Joint Commission on Accreditation of Healthcare Organizations has now stipulated that any laboratory test result that requires a telephone report, for example, to report a critically abnormal result, requires 'read back' from the recipient to confirm that the message has been accurately communicated.

The rule is simple: when receiving a telephone communication regarding a test result, 'read back' the name of the patient, the test, and the test result to the message sender to confirm that you have received the correct information. When giving a test result, ask the message recipient to 'read back' the information you have just relayed to them.

It seems so easy and so sensible to apply 'read back' in many other situations in healthcare.

Simple 'read back'

Simple 'read back' is where the message recipient repeats back exactly the same words used by the sender. This is also known as 'parroting' (that is repeating back 'parrot fashion').

In most straightforward situations this is usually adequate. This 'simple read back' procedure is successfully used hundreds of thousands of times world-wide each day by pilots when receiving instructions from air traffic control. Although 'simple read back' generally substantially improves the reliability of verbal SCCs, on *very* rare occasions there can still be a misunderstanding.

The reasons for these 'read back' failures include:

- The message sender makes a slip of the tongue when uttering the message in the first place and, while the other party's 'read back' represents a faithful reproduction of the words actually uttered, the sender fails to notice that the 'read back' does not reflect what he had actually intended to say. (> Sender's fault.)

- The receiver mishears or misunderstands the message and in a second error, the sender fails to notice that the receiver has not 'read back' correctly. (> Receiver's and sender's fault.) This double failure is the cause of the relatively few catastrophic failures in communications between air traffic control and pilots.

- The receiver 'parrots' back the message correctly without really under-standing it or appreciating its significance or all of its implications. (> Receiver's fault.)

- The receiver mishears the message, reads back incorrectly and then terminates the conversation (e.g. puts down the telephone) before the sender has the opportunity to confirm that the 'read back' is correct. (> Receiver's fault.) This last event is what happened in case study 12 (in Chapter 4).

Most of these problems can usually be mitigated by the use of the 'enhanced' form of 'read back' described in the paragraphs below.

Paraphrased (reworded) 'read back'

In paraphrased 'read back', the message receiver listens to the message, takes a moment to understand it and then constructs a 'read back' using different words of the same meaning. Alternatively he might change the word order slightly while retaining the essence of the message. He may add an appropriate brief phrase to reflect his understanding of the background of the communication or to enhance the communication process generally.

Another advantage of this type of 'read back' is that, in paraphrasing the message, the receiver may also consider potential problems when implementing any instructions contained in the message.

In this way the problems that were described above in relation to 'simple read back', may be overcome. The sender will notice that the receiver is not merely parroting back the message and, therefore, he has to 'actively listen' in order to ensure that the reworded version matches the essence of the original.

Paraphrased 'read back' is likely to be particularly useful in healthcare where the complexity of clinical situations mean that range of potential misunderstandings is much greater than in those 'safety-critical' industries where operational conditions are much less complex. Paraphrased 'read back' can also improve the communication of subtleties, which are important in many of the 'grey areas' of clinical practice.

> *Doctor A*: 'When the CT scan comes back if it shows intracerebral haemorrhage, reverse the warfarin with FFP and intravenous vitamin K and recheck the clotting.'
>
> *Doctor B*: 'OK if it's a bleed I will reverse the warfarin and I will recheck the clotting'.
>
> *Doctor A*: 'Yes that is correct'.

'Read back': pronouns

When articulating the 'read back' it is important to replace any pronouns (he, him, she, her, it) with the actual name of the patient or medication, route, etc.

> *Sender*: 'OK give it to him'
>
> *Receiver*: 'OK—just to double check I'll give 40 mg i.v. of furosemide to Brian Royle immediately'
>
> *Sender*: 'Yes that is correct'.

Identifying the parties to the communication

It is not difficult to imagine how the passing or receiving of messages/instructions to or from the wrong person can be very hazardous.

In order to mitigate these risks, SCC protocols require a robust identification process if there is any possibility of misidentification before the main part of the message is passed. In most SCC protocols the sender identifies himself first. This is followed by the name of the intended addressee.

The issues related to misidentification of patients are covered in Chapter 2.

Clear diction and use of 'standard English'

Consider these two situations:

1 Approximately 8% of the population is either deaf or hard of hearing. In the age group 55–64 years, this percentage increases to 15%.

2 Each year more clinicians whose first language is not English join the NHS. Each year more patients whose first language is not English require treatment.

For these and other reasons, the use of clear diction and 'standard English' enhances safe communication.

Recordings of conversations in safety-critical industries show that people often start speaking spontaneously without first having taken an adequate breath. As a result the opening syllables of the message are inadequately voiced and the latter part of the message may 'tail off' as a result of lack of breath. Most of the time we do not notice this because the context and body language enable us to unconsciously infer the missing elements. It is possible, for example, that a message such as 'I'm not sure if **he's had the antibiotics**' might be perceived as '... he's had the antibiotics'.

Modern culture favours slick verbal interactions. Railway managers, auditing recordings of SCC in their industry, noticed the occasional use of a casual verbal style they referred to as 'matespeak'. This might be appropriate for a group of mates in a pub but not for SCC.

There is a tendency to use 'hip' phrases or words. For example, the phrase 'Is there any chance of ...?' is often nowadays used to introduce a request. A person whose first language is not English might not understand that this is a request and might think that the action mentioned has already been carried out.

There is also a tendency to affect a 'fashionable' accent, such as the unpretentious Essex dialect 'estuary English'. These tendencies may adversely affect the intelligibility of the message particularly among the growing proportion of clinicians whose first language is not English.

Thus, SCC should use 'standard English'.

One should emulate the delivery of the BBC news readers!

Opening phrases/alert phrases

Most people speak at the rate of 60–80 words per minute. However, we are able to listen and understand at the rate of 100–120 words per minute.

There is a critical mismatch here. We are able to mentally process an incoming verbal message at a rate greater than it is being received. This produces a tendency in many people to 'jump ahead' and try to guess how the message will end. There may be a subconscious tendency where we actually think we have heard someone say what we expected them to say.

Thus there can be a problem when a message begins with what seems to be a routine introduction but then contains a later element that differs significantly from that which might be expected. In this case the message receiver may fail to notice the crucial difference.

Another problem can occur when the message sender uses a 'normal' tone for an urgent, abnormal, or emergency message. The receiver may assume that the message is routine and not give the message the special attention that it requires.

One solution to this problem can lie in the use of an 'opening phrase'. For example, when air traffic controllers have to give an instruction that differs from normal practice, they begin their message with the words 'This is non-standard, ….' This alerts the pilot to the potential for a misunderstanding in the message that follows.

> The fatal adverse event in case study 12 might have been avoided if the path lab technician had opened his message with the phrase: 'This is an abnormal result'.

Railway safety officials, studying recordings of safety-critical telephone and radio communications have noticed that when the message sender sets the right tone by starting with a clear opening phrase, the receiver will usually adopt safe communication behaviours as well:

> A communication that begins 'safely' will usually continue in that way.

Alert phrases

Investigations into many accidents in 'safety-critical' domains, including healthcare, have revealed that one or more members of the operational team were aware that something was going wrong. Frustratingly, this recognition occurred at a time when it was still possible to reverse those errors that had already been made. Unfortunately, the team's attention was not drawn to the fact that they were observing the symptoms of an incipient adverse event.

A growing number of high reliability organizations believe that it is important to formally institute certain phrases, known as 'alert phrases', which are intended to be used by team members who believe that they have noticed uncertainties or errors in the operational situation and who wish to draw their unease to the attention of the team (in Chapter 5 we have already discussed the equivalent system of PACE used in the airline industry). These alert phrases are universally recognized throughout the organization as an indication of impending error.

These phrases, which are written into the organization's official procedures manuals, can also help with the problem of the tongue-tied operator who needs to say something but does not know what to say or how to introduce his comment.

> In using an alert phrase, he is saying: 'Something may be wrong, I'm not sure what it is. Rather than allowing this operation to continue while I try to accurately describe what I fear may be happening, I think we should stop now and we should all reassess the situation'.

The Allina Hospital Group[12] in the USA has introduced the following 'alert phrase' for its personnel who encounter uncertainty in their work:

'I need some clarity here ...'

Many airlines suggest/require their pilots to use the following 'alert phrases'

'I think we have some red flags here,...'

'I am not happy,...'

'I am uncomfortable ...'

'You must listen,...'

Conditional phrases

The following advice may sound obvious but there is evidence from some organizations with advanced safety cultures that it is still not always being followed. Recently, following an audit of radio messages, the UK air traffic control service has had to issue a bulletin to controllers and pilots to remind them of the following rule.

> Where an instruction depends upon a condition (if/when event 'X' occurs, carry out action 'Y'), the condition must be stated first, in the opening phrase:
>
> Example:
>
> 'If the urine output falls below 50 ml/hour, give a fluid challenge of 500 mls of normal saline'
>
> Note that if the message is passed in this sequence:
>
> 'Give a fluid challenge of 500 mls of normal saline, if the urine output falls below 50 ml/hour'

and the second part of the message is distorted or suppressed by extraneous noise or other disturbance then a hazardous misunderstanding may take place.

REMEMBER, condition first, instruction second

Standard words/message structures/sequences of data

On occasions where a large amount of data has to be communicated on a regular basis, it can be safer to transmit the data in a standardized sequence. Once personnel are familiar with the sequence any errors and missing elements are much more likely to be detected.

Recently, the Royal College of Surgeons have suggested that surgical procedures should be described in the sequence SITE/OPERATION/SIDE. For example, kidney, nephrectomy, right.

As subspecialization becomes increasingly common in healthcare, more and more patients are going to transfer, temporarily or otherwise, from one department to another. No patient should leave one department for another without adequate documentation communicating all of their vital clinical information in a standardized format.

Use the NATO phonetic code

Much communication in healthcare takes place using the telephone. One problem that affects intelligibility of telephone conversations is the available sound 'bandwidth'. Human speech usually covers a 'bandwidth' (frequency range) of about 9 kHz. The range starts at about 1 kHz—for deep male voices up to about 10 kHz—for the best reproduction of consonants. The reception of consonants is crucial to intelligibility.

Telephones, however, are generally limited to a 2 kHz bandwidth, and this makes it hard to distinguish between high-pitched consonant sounds, particularly 'f' and 's' or 'd' and 't' sounds. We may remember spelling names over the telephone and having difficulty in achieving understanding of 'eff'/'ess' and 'dee'/'tee'. The numbers 5 and 9 have the same vowel sound and, with their consonants suppressed, can sound very similar over the telephone (f *a* i v, n *a* i n).

To prevent such misunderstandings, most high reliability organizations use the NATO code to spell out names over the telephone and the radio.

The NATO code is used by many national and international organizations, including NHS Ambulance Trusts (see box below if you might want to consider using the NATO phonetic code).

NATO phonetic code

A—Alpha	J—Juliett	S—Sierra	The numbers are the same
B—Bravo	K—Kilo	T—Tango	except that the following
C—Charlie	L—Lima	U—Uniform	are pronounced thus:
D—Delta	M—Mike	V—Victor	
E—Echo	N—November	W—Whiskey	3—'tree'
F—Foxtrot	O—Oscar	X—X-ray	5—'fife'
G—Golf	P—Papa	Y—Yankee	9—'niner'
H—Hotel	Q—Quebec	Z—Zulu	0—zero
I—India	R—Romeo		decimal point—'dayseemal'

Avoiding: non-pertinent communication/communicating at an inappropriate time/abbreviations/non-standard terminology

Several cockpit voice recordings from crashed aircraft showed that the pilots were having a discussion of non-pertinent matters in the moments just before the accident and it was clear that these communications fatally distracted the pilots. As a result airlines insist on a 'sterile cockpit' rule that prohibits non-pertinent communications during high-risk periods of a flight, such as take-off and landing.

Case study

A man of about 40 came into a GP's evening surgery. The previous day he had slipped and fallen down a small flight of stairs. He had been able to walk immediately after the accident and thus thought he had only mildly sprained his ankle. However, the ankle pain had not got better afterwards.

During their opening conversation the patient and the GP happened to discover that, most remarkably, they had an unexpected mutual acquaintance. The GP then examined the patient, but could find no positive signs apart from the swelling. The conversation about the mutual friend then resumed for several minutes. The GP finished by giving the patient some advice about support and exercise for a sprained ankle.

A few weeks later, the patient went to A&E because he was still in pain. An X-ray showed a fractured fibula at the ankle, which the GP had missed. The fracture had mis-united because he had been walking on it and an open reduction of the fracture was subsequently required.

> In hindsight, the GP believes that the conversation about their mutual acquaintance had distracted him from carrying out an adequate examination and organizing an X-ray.

When you are about to initiate a communication take a moment to assess whether your message is important enough to justify interrupting the intended receiver if they are busy.

In the Piper Alpha case (p. 155), the engineer made the wrong decision, he should have interrupted. In other cases delaying the communication might be wise.

An example (which happens frequently) occurs when asking the anaesthetist to give the pre-operative prophylactic antibiotics. We know from our own audit of administration of pre-operative antibiotic prophylaxis that in 10% of cases appropriate antibiotic prophylaxis is not given simply because both the surgeon and the anaesthetist just forget.

There are several reasons for this, but one reason is failure to ask the anaesthetist to give the antibiotics at a time when the anaesthetist is likely to be receptive to your request. Asking the anaesthetist to give the prophylactic antibiotics when he is dealing with a difficult airways problem is not sensible. In his anxious struggle to secure the airways, it is *very* unlikely that the anaesthetist will hear your request and even if he does hear you, he will certainly have a more pressing situation on his hands to deal with and certainly won't comply with your request then and there.

When the 'excitement' of managing the airways is over, it is likely that he will have forgotten your request for prophylactic antibiotics and as a consequence they will never be given. So, the timing of your communication is *critical* to the likelihood that it will be a successful communication.

On other occasions **non-standard terminology** has contributed to errors.

In the USA, the National Coordinating Council for Medication Error Reporting and Prevention (NCC MERP) has issued a list of terminology and abbreviations that have been associated with medication errors. On their web-site[13] they have a list of recommended terminology and abbreviations.

Problems include:

- µg intended to mean micrograms was misread as mg (milligrams). This resulted in an overdose.
- 4.0 mg was misread as 40 mg. As a result the NCC MERP suggests that the trailing zero should not be used, e.g. 4 mg. In the same way half a milligram should be written as 0.5 mg (and not as .5 mg).

- ◆ Q.D., the Latin abbreviation for 'every day' has been misread as QiD, 'four times' a day.
- ◆ SC—subcutaneous was misread as SL sublingual due to poor handwriting.

There are many more examples.

Awareness of communication failure scenarios

Each of the individual SCC protocols that have been adopted in high reliability industries are the direct result of lessons learned from one or more major adverse events. It is important that personnel are made aware in some detail of the circumstances of these events. In this way they are more likely to accept the need for and comply with these communication procedures.

Having knowledge of a wide range of adverse event case studies, personnel are able to interpolate between them and consider other circumstances that may not have caused accidents in the past but may do in the future. As a result they can apply this awareness to the way they formulate safety-critical messages.

Types of error according to communication method

- ◆ Verbal—face to face
    - —failure to identify the parties to the communication
    - —poor diction
    - —inappropriate body language
    - —lack of alert phrases or other relevant opening phrases
    - —failure to get to the point
- ◆ Verbal—telephone conversation
    - —failure to identify the parties to the communication
    - —lack of alert phrases or other relevant opening phrases
    - —poor diction
    - —reduced sound bandwidth
    - —misheard spellings
    - —failure to get to the point
- ◆ Pager
    - —paging the wrong person
    - —assuming because you have paged someone they will or are in a position to reply (the 'paged' person may be on leave)

- Written—entries made in hospital notes
  —poor handwriting
  —writing in the wrong set of notes
  —multiple sets of notes
- Fax
  —the fax number may be wrong
  —the fax machine may be out of paper
  —the staff who 'attend' the fax machine may be away
  —the doctor for whom the fax is intended is on leave.
- Email
  —'emailed' person may, for example, be on leave and might have forgotten to switch on their 'out of office' auto reply.
- Internet.

How to prevent communication errors in specific healthcare situations

In addition to the use of the general protocols given above the following may enhance effective communication in various specific healthcare situations and prevent communication errors in healthcare:

- summing up discussions
- handovers
- briefings
- communicating concerns about a patient's condition
- avoiding the use of ambiguous abbreviations.

Summing up discussions

In healthcare there are numerous discussions in which a number of management options for a patient are discussed. These discussions may result in a change in the treatment plan.

In many adverse event case studies it has been noted that, when two clinicians parted after a discussion, their subsequent actions strongly suggested that they had divergent understandings of what they thought they had agreed. This result could have been prevented if one party had taken a moment to 'summarize' the final plan:

'So, to sum up, the plan is now ... '

or

'So, to sum up, the plan has changed from ... And is now ... '

A commonly occurring problem, particularly where there is a change of plan, is the failure of the team to positively allocate a given task to an individual. People often assume that someone else is going to carry out a task. Thus it is important that the 'summer-up' specifies precisely who does what.

Example

Message

Doctor A: 'Mr Smith needs his pulse and blood pressure checking every hour for the next 12 hours. Make sure the urine output is monitored every hour and if it falls below 50 ml/hour give a fluid challenge of 500 ml of normal saline. Make sure the haemoglobin and U&Es are checked first thing in the morning and let me know the result by early afternoon. OK?'

Summary

Doctor B: '**So, to sum up**, I'm going to monitor the pulse and blood pressure every hour over the next 12 hours. The urine output also needs to be checked every hour. If it falls below 50 ml/hour I'll give a fluid challenge of 500 ml of normal saline. I'll check the haemoglobin and U&Es first thing in the morning and let you know the result by early afternoon. Have I got all of that correct?'

Doctor A: 'Yes that is all correct'.

Handovers between shifts

Handovers between shifts can be highly productive of serious communication failures. The Piper Alpha oil rig and Chernobyl nuclear power station disasters were initiated when information was not passed between shifts.

A medical or surgical handover can be defined as 'the transfer of professional responsibility and accountability for some or all aspects of care for a patient, or group of patients, to another person or professional group on a temporary or permanent basis'.[14]

In the days when teams of doctors worked for continuous periods of 24 hours or longer, there were fewer points at which the handover of safety-critical information was necessary. In order to avoid excessive hours on duty when exhausted doctors were expected to perform safely there has been a steady and welcome reduction in the length of time a doctor may remain on duty without a break. Reduced working periods and the move towards shift-based working consequent upon the European Working Time Directive has resulted in more a frequent requirement for handovers between teams.

The following example highlights the problems that can occur when the handover system does not 'handover' effectively.

A 56-year-old woman was admitted as an emergency in the early hours of the morning with breathlessness and weakness following a few days of vomiting. A number of 'routine' investigations were performed by the night team, one of which was a serum calcium concentration that turned out to be extremely low. The result was available online but was not flagged by the biochemistry department nor was the ward or the doctor in charge informed. When the morning team took over the incoming junior doctor saw the result on the computer but because it was the lowest such value he had seen he repeated the test thinking there had been some sort of laboratory error. The result of this repeat test was available mid afternoon and again it was dangerously low, but there was no record that the laboratory had contacted any clinical staff involved in the patient's care and they remained unaware.

The woman had improved somewhat in the afternoon and no one appears to have actively sought out the repeat result. When the evening shift team took over they were unaware that there was a repeat test outstanding so they did not actively look out for it. 16 hours after admission the woman experienced breathing difficulties and died an hour later. After a post mortem examination the cause of death was given as hypocalcaemia.

This case illustrates a number of systematic failures in communication:

- If you request an investigation it is your responsibility to seek out the result or pass on to the next team the fact that there are investigations outstanding.
- Never assume an abnormal result is a laboratory error without first checking with the laboratory itself.
- Many hospitals work with systems where laboratory results are available online very rapidly but this requires someone to access the results and to be aware that they are outstanding. Dangerously abnormal results should also be flagged with the medical team in charge. This makes it essential that the laboratory staff know who is in charge and how to contact them.

Handover arrangements between teams clearly failed in this instance, three separate teams were involved in 16 hours and yet none appreciated that there were results on the computer system that could have resulted in a simple and life-saving intervention.

You should take 'lead responsibility' for any investigation that you request. Always make an entry in the notes stating which investigations you have requested and at the end of your shift always ensure you have checked and documented all of the investigations you have requested. If any result is outstanding then the team taking over needs to be aware that they need to chase this up.

Handover methods

♦ Verbal only

♦ Verbal with note taking

♦ Verbal with pre-prepared information sheet containing all relevant patient details

♦ Telephone handover.

Bhabra *et al*.'s group from Bristol[15] tested the percentage of data points (single facts of variable importance to patient safety) retained by doctors using various handover techniques. The percentage of information retained over five handover cycles (handover between five consecutive doctors) was:

♦ Verbal only: 2.5%

♦ Verbal with note taking: 85.5%

♦ Verbal with pre-prepared information sheet containing all relevant patient details 99%.

Thus, very few facts are retained by a verbal-only method of handover. Handover techniques that use note taking or written information sheets result in a far greater degree of retention of safety-critical information. Handover using a printed sheet requires regular updating of the information by an individual, and on a busy ward this may not always be practical.

In the Department of Urology in Oxford we have instituted a system of handovers between teams that involves a combination of verbal with note taking and face-to-face patient to doctor consultation, with the 'day team' physically taking the 'night team' to the bedside of patients with ongoing problems, so that the handover is done in front of the patient. The 'night team' writes down safety-critical points so that these may be referred back to as and when required.

The same system operates when the 'night team' hands over to the 'day team'.

Our medical teams in Oxford, who look after much larger numbers of patients, formally hand over safety-critical information from the evening to night team. This process involves both teams meeting and handing over information directly. A consultant leads this handover.

Specific safety-critical times of potential communication failure: the special case of change of personnel during a surgical operation

From time to time, particularly during long surgical operations, the scrub nurse who started the case will hand over to a new scrub nurse. This can be a point at which an error of a retained instrument or swab is generated. A communication failure is the root cause of many incidents of retained foreign bodies.

During changes of personnel during surgical operations, as the operating surgeon insists that the two nurses who change places do a combined swab and instrument count before they hand over.

> Changes of personnel during operations (specifically the 'scrub' nurse) is a cause of retained instruments or swabs. Insist on a swab and instrument count before the two nurses hand over.

Pre-procedure briefings/checklist

The Toronto study into verbal communications in the operating room[3] found that 30% of the communications between members of the surgical team 'failed'. A third of these failures resulted in effects that jeopardized patient safety. The report of the study suggested that 'the current weaknesses in communication in the operating theatre may derive from a lack of standardization and team integration'.

One potential solution suggested in the report is to adapt the briefing and checklist system currently in use in aviation for pre-flight team communications. This briefing and checklist system structures the communication of critical information to ensure that team members possess all of the data they need for their work. The timing of this process allows the cross-checking of the data to take place before safety-critical activities commence. In this way the correction of problems can be made when they will not cause hazardous distractions to members of the team.

While there are obvious differences between an operating theatre and an aircraft cockpit, the report's authors anticipate that a carefully adapted checklist system could promote safer, more effective communications in the operating theatre team.

There is evidence[16] that pre-procedure briefings:

- enhance situation awareness across the whole surgical team (e.g. between anaesthetist, scrub nurses, and surgeon), making all staff more aware of which patient they should be operating on, what operation they are going to do, and for lateralized procedures, which side they are going to operate on
- promote more effective team-working between surgeons, anaesthetists, and operating theatre staff.

Impact of pre-procedure briefings on wrong side surgery

The major cause of wrong site and wrong side surgery is a failure of communication between members of the surgical team.

Makary et al.[16] has stated that the low frequency of wrong site and wrong side surgery 'makes it logistically difficult to evaluate the effectiveness of interventions designed to prevent wrong-site surgery', but there is at least

- ◆ What are the **names and roles** of the team members?
- ◆ Is the correct patient/procedure confirmed?
- ◆ Have **antibiotics** been given?
- ◆ What are the **critical steps** of the procedure?
- ◆ What are the **potential problems** for the case?

Fig. 6.1 A pre-procedure briefing tool (checklists) (adapted from Makary 2007).

a *perception* among members of operating theatre teams that pre-procedure briefings reduce the risk of wrong side surgery.

Various checklists have been developed as a means of allowing members of the operating team to reduce the chance of wrong procedure, wrong site, and wrong side operation (as well as to ensure that appropriate thromboembolic prevention and antibiotic prophylaxis has been administered). Fig. 6.1 shows a pre-procedure briefing tool (checklist) (adapted from Makary *et al.*[16]) and see Fig. 7.7 for another pre-procedure checklist that is used in the Department of Urology in Oxford in the operating theatre; the anaesthetist and urologist complete this second checklist when the patient has been stabilized on the operating table prior to commencement of the surgical scrub. This can be done in under 60 seconds.

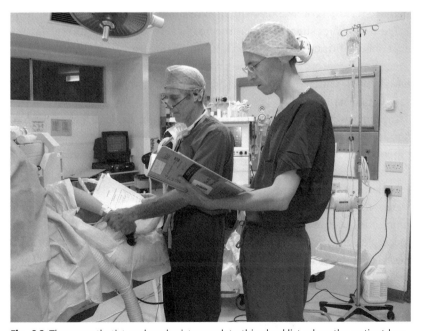

Fig. 6.2 The anaesthetist and urologist complete this checklist when the patient has been stabilized on the operating table, before commencing the surgical scrub. This can be done in under 60 seconds.

The major cause of wrong site and wrong side surgery is a failure of communication between members of the surgical team. Pre-procedure briefings reduce the risk of wrong side surgery.

Communicating concerns about a patient's condition

The Kaiser Permanente Hospital Group in the USA noticed[17] that it had had a significant number of cases where patients had died following a 'failure of recognition and rescue' by their clinicians. It seemed that the conditions of many patients had deteriorated without experienced doctors attending.

They found that the causes of these failures fell into two main types.

1 Failure to recognize the patient was in trouble.

2 Failure to rescue—reluctance of nurses and junior doctors to communicate with senior doctors to call for help:

   ◆ senior doctors not accepting the urgency of the situation
   ◆ incomplete data communicated.

The first element was dealt with by improving clinical training. With respect to the second element, the hospital's patient safety trainers approached a university that had research connections with high reliability organizations.

The academics suggested that the hospital trainers should consider the experience of trainers of naval officers on US nuclear-powered submarines. These naval officers have to undertake regular training exercises where they have to work under acute time pressures to resolve a simulated crisis with the vessels' nuclear reactor.

Information to help the team to diagnose and deal with the problem has to be passed rapidly between team members. These exercises are video-taped and afterwards the exercises are analysed by trainers and the teams are debriefed.

In those cases where the crisis was not well handled it was noted that things started to go wrong very early in the exercise. This was because the first communications between team members about the problems with the reactor were incomplete or elements of the message were not given the right emphasis. This necessitated further communications to clarify certain points and this, in turn, delayed effective remedial measures.

It became clear that the teams needed a simple protocol to help them formulate accurate and complete *initial* messages. In an iterative process the trainers tried out a number sequences of data before they settled on the SBAR protocol.

> **SBAR** = situation, background, assessment, recommendation. Data about the problem was sequenced in that order.

The teams then had training courses where they practised passing messages using this protocol. After 30 minutes or so team members found that they had mastered the art of structuring their messages into the SBAR sequence.

When the simulated reactor crisis exercises were re-run the performance of the teams was significantly improved. When completely new teams were trained in SBAR before they had carried any simulated exercises, their performance was significantly better than those who had not had the SBAR training.

The Kaiser Permanente Patient Safety Trainers were impressed by the effectiveness of SBAR and they adapted it for use in their hospitals. An initial 'I' for identification was added to ensure the parties are talking about the correct patient.

Other healthcare organizations in the USA have started to train clinicians to use ISBAR.

In both the navy and in the hospital setting, role-play exercises are used to carry out training in the use of ISBAR.

ISBAR report: Example

Identification

'Mr Lenham, this is Peter, I'm calling about Mr Grantham, who had a colectomy earlier today … '

Situation

'I've just assessed the situation. His blood pressure is 80 over 50 and his pulse is 140'.

Background

'The background is that we've given 2 units of blood and 2 units of gelofusine, but despite this his blood pressure has not responded … '

Assessment

'My assessment is that he's bleeding (or—I am not sure what the problem is but the patient is deteriorating …)'.

Recommendation

'I think he needs a laparotomy—could you come and see him to check that you agree?'

Checklist/aide memoire SBAR report about a critical situation

Situation

I am calling about <**patient name and location**>.

The patient's code status is <**code status**>

The problem I am calling about is _____.

I am afraid the patient is going to arrest.

I have just assessed the patient personally:

Vital signs are: Blood pressure _____/_____, Pulse _____, Respiration_____ and temperature _____

I am concerned about the:

- Blood pressure because it is over 200 or less than 100 or 30 mmHg below usual
- Pulse because it is over 140 or less than 50
- Respiration because it is less than 5 or over 40.
- Temperature because it is less than 96 or over 104.

Background

The patient's mental status is:

- Alert and oriented to person place and time.
- Confused and cooperative or non-cooperative
- Agitated or combative
- Lethargic but conversant and able to swallow
- Stuporous and not talking clearly and possibly not able to swallow
- Comatose. Eyes closed. Not responding to stimulation.

The skin is:

- Warm and dry
- Pale
- Mottled
- Extremities are cold
- Extremities are warm

The patient is not or is on oxygen.

The patient has been on _____ (l/min) or (%) oxygen for _____ minutes (hours)

The oximeter is reading _____%

The oximeter does not detect a good pulse and is giving erratic readings.

Assessment

This is what I think the problem is: <say what you think is the problem>

The problem seems to be cardiac/infective/neurological/respiratory, etc. _____

I am not sure what the problem is but the patient is deteriorating.

The patient seems to be unstable and may get worse, we need to do something.

Recommendation

I suggest or request that you <say what you would like to see done>.

- transfer the patient to critical care
- come to see the patient at this time.
- talk to the patient or family about code status.
- ask the on-call family practice resident to see the patient now.
- ask for a consultant to see the patient now.

Are any tests needed:

- Do you need any tests like CXR, ABG, ECG, FBC?
- Others?

If a change in treatment is ordered then ask:

- How often do you want vital signs?
- How long to you expect this problem will last?
- If the patient does not get better when would you want us to call again?

Examples of SBAR in use:

- *Situation*: Dr Jones, I'm Paul, the respiratory therapist. There's someone downstairs who's in serious respiratory distress.
- *Background*: he has severe COPD, has been going downhill, and is now acutely worse. RR 40, O_2 sats 74%.
- *Assessment*: his breath sounds are way down on the right side ... I think he has a pneumothorax and needs a chest tube pronto before he stops breathing.
- *Recommendation*: I really need your help now ... this guy's in real trouble.

- *Situation*: Dr Samet, this is Lisa Williamson, I'm worried about Mrs Artan. I think she's going to rupture her uterus.
- *Background*: she has a dense epidural, but is having persistent break-through abdominal pain; she's completely dilated and ready to push.
- *Assessment*: I'm concerned—something's wrong—I don't want her to push.
- *Recommendation*: I think we need to think about a C-section. I need you to come see her now.

Communicating with patients

Avoid the use of euphemisms

Doctors sometimes use a variety of terms to hide what they really mean, often out of a misguided desire not to hurt a patient's feelings. Bladder cancer is a good example of this. Bladder tumours, which usually present with haematuria, have been variously described as 'polyps', 'warts', 'trouble in the bladder', 'growths', 'sea anemones', or 'mushrooms', a whole host of alternatives to the simple, but very clear word 'cancer'. These terms are used out of a desire not to upset people. However, such attempts are misguided, because they can lull patients into a false sense of security. The haematuria in such patients is often intermittent and so when it resolves the patient is reassured that all is well, and this false sense of well-being is reinforced by the use of terms such as 'wart' or 'mushroom'. After all, no one *dies* as a consequence of 'warts' or 'mushrooms', but patients certainly die from bladder cancer, which is often a highly aggressive disease, curable only by prompt diagnosis and treatment.

So, if you mean 'cancer', use the term 'cancer'. Do not beat about the bush. The use of the term can be communicated with compassion, but it must be communicated.

Avoiding ambiguous abbreviations

The use of ambiguous abbreviations in verbal and written communications (e.g. medical notes) can create the risk of serious errors. The Medical Defence Union said difficulties often arise because abbreviations can have more than one meaning or might be misread.

A recent US study of 30 000 medication errors showed 5% were linked to abbreviations of drug names, dosages, or the frequency of administration. Some of these errors had fatal consequences.

One example involved a 62-year-old patient on haemodialysis who was treated for a viral infection with the drug acyclovir. The order for acyclovir was written as 'acyclovir (unknown dose) with HD', meaning haemodialysis.

Acyclovir should be adjusted for renal impairment and given only once daily. Unfortunately, the order was misread as TID (three times daily) and the patient died as a result.

A UK audit by the paediatric department at Birmingham Heartlands Hospital, published in the *Archives of Disease in Childhood*, found instances where abbreviations used had caused confusion because they had multiple interpretations. For example, 'TOF' could be taken to mean 'Tetralogy of Fallot' or 'tracheo-oesophageal fistula'—two completely different conditions.

When presented with a selection of abbreviations, the study authors found paediatric doctors agreed on the interpretation of 56–94% of the abbreviations while other healthcare professionals recognized only 31–63%. The authors also found that the use of abbreviations was inconsistent—15% of the abbreviations used in medical notes appeared in the hospital's intranet dictionary while 17% appeared in a medical dictionary used by paediatric secretaries.

The MDU, which defends members' reputations when their clinical performance is called into question, advises doctors to use only the abbreviations or acronyms that are unambiguous and approved in their practice or hospital.

Composing an 'abnormal' (non-routine) safety-critical message

Messages that come 'out of the blue'

Most 'safety-critical' communications occur in a context where the receiver can safely infer the purpose of the message and any missing message elements.

Sometimes, however, abnormal circumstances may require the message sender to initiate a communication that will be received by the receiver, so to speak, 'out of the blue'. The receiver may thus not be able to instantly deduce the context or importance of the message. Thus they might be unable to infer any missing elements or understand the urgency of the message.

If you study the adverse event case reports you will see that in a significant proportion of cases they involved a misunderstanding about one of the following situations:

- Sudden/unexpected deterioration of a patient's condition
- Unusual patient conditions, such as abnormal anatomy
- Changes of plan, such as the order of patients on an operating list:
  —change of diagnosis
  —change of treatment plan
  —change of personnel to carry out a procedure.

The following approach might help you to communicate safely in these potentially hazardous situations:

> ## STOP—THINK—ARTICULATE—READ BACK

Stop

Stop for a moment.

> Remember that a misunderstood communication about a patient can be as harmful as a misdiagnosis or a medication error.

Except in very rare fast-moving crisis events there is almost always time for a brief moment of thought and mental preparation. If necessary you can say 'Please stand by for a moment'.

On the positive side, a timely, well structured verbal communication about a patient's treatment can mark a positive turning point. This is particularly true if the message:

- identifies a neglected issue
- defines an uncertainty
- summarizes a discussion.

Think

Junior doctors often feel under pressure to speak spontaneously so as to appear 'sharp' and efficient in the presence of their seniors. Thus they may make, unknowingly or knowingly, an erroneous statement. They may plan to correct any knowingly incorrect remark later. Fortunately for the patient the senior doctor can sometimes detect such a erroneous statement, having been a junior once themselves ('Have you really arranged that test?'). In the UK's last major air disaster in 1989 the co-pilot appears to have contributed to the event by announcing a quick but tragically flawed diagnosis of the engine problem.

In his book entitled *Assert Yourself*, Robert Sharp[18] argues that pausing before replying to another's question or remark helps one to be more assertive. In confrontation situations, he notes that the other party is often confounded if you pause before replying. It seems that if the other party knows that his line of reasoning is not a strong one, he may feel the need to fill the silence with further remarks. These additional remarks may be ill judged, offering the opportunity to correct any weakness in his position.

When you are about to initiate a communication take a moment to assess whether your message is important enough to justify interrupting the intended receiver if they are busy.

Think about the type of message you want to send—Is it a request, an instruction or a piece of data, or an expression of unease about a situation?

Think, ask yourself the following questions:
- Is this the **right time** to send this message?
- Are you addressing the **right person**?
- What is the **right medium** for this message?
- Do you have all of the **relevant data** to hand? Is it accurate data?
- Do you need to use an **opening phrase** that makes the purpose of the message absolutely clear?
- Would it be helpful to compose the message using one of the following structures?
  NEED/DATA/ACTION (for general messages)
  SBAR (for messages about a patient's condition)
- Consider how your message could possibly be misunderstood—*be risk conscious*

Articulate

- Take a breath so that you are able to voice the entire message clearly.
- If possible, make eye contact with the other party.
- Using the other party's name is usually helpful. It will help to engage their attention.
- Use straight-forward words. Avoid the use of abbreviations, esoteric terminology.

Response/read back

Observe how the message is received, particularly the body language of the receiver. Listen to the read back.

If there is any doubt that the message has been successfully passed, re-send the message using different words or message structure.

Opening phrase/alert phrase

Use an opening phrase or an alert phrase if appropriate. Examples can include those shown in Table 6.1.

Table 6.1 Examples of opening and alert phrases

Opening phrases	Alert phrases
'Please stand by for a moment'	'I need a little clarity ...'
'I have a request. ...'	'I think we have some red flags here, ...'
'This is an emergency...'	'I could not help noticing that...'
'This is an abnormal test result ...'	'I need to understand why ...'
'This is urgent...'	'I am not happy about this...'
'This is a change of plan...'	'I am concerned...'
'This is non-standard...'	'I am uncomfortable ...'
'This is not what you are expecting, but...'	'Something's wrong...'
'This is a correction...'	'You must listen...'
'This is to sum up...'	'STOP NOW'
'This is a safety-critical message'	

Need/data/action

It might be useful for the message sender to pause for a moment, where possible, and take the time to construct the message using the sequence:

NEED, DATA, ACTION

Successful messages of this type should contain at least two and, possibly all three, of these elements. Where an instruction has to be given it might be helpful to give the 'need' that the instruction addresses as well as the required action: NEED–ACTION.

Need (purpose)

All 'safety-critical' messages are intended to address some need or purpose:

- Someone needs someone else to do something.
- Someone needs to give or receive some information.
- Someone needs to express their unease about something.

Communication can be enhanced if the message sender states explicitly exactly what purpose the communication is intended to address. If you are in doubt as to the purpose of your message is, try starting a sentence with one of the following:

I need...

We need ...

You need …

The patient needs …

By the time you have uttered these words **what the need is** may have become clearer to you. For example:

I need… to let you know about a deterioration in Mr Andrew Robinson's condition …

We need … to have another discussion about Mrs Gregson's diagnosis.

Data

Ensure that any data in your message are as accurate as possible. Before initiating a message about a patient it might be helpful to ensure that you have valid data available. You should ask yourself the following questions:

- Have I seen and assessed the patient myself before initiating this message?
- Has the situation been discussed with other clinicians?
- Review the notes so you can decide who the most appropriate physician to call is.
- Know the admitting diagnosis and date of admission.
- Have I read the most recent notes and notes from the doctor who worked the shift ahead of me?
- Do I have available the following items when communicating:
  —patient's observation chart with blood pressure, pulse, urine, and drain outputs
  —list of current medications, allergies, intravenous fluids, and test results
  —reporting lab results: provide the date and time test was done and results ofprevious tests for comparison
  —code status

Note: There may be no data about a particular aspect of the patient's condition. One of the case studies in this handbook (p. 244) involved a patient misidentification where one doctor recognized the absence of relevant data in the (wrong) patient's notes. Thus the fact that there are 'no data' is the 'data'.

Action

Some communications fail because the sender does not clearly state what the receiver is expected to do with the data. Usually this is obvious but in many cases it can be useful to state it.

Several adverse event case studies have resulted from flawed assumptions that someone else was going to carry out an action. In healthcare, demarcation of work roles is not always adequately defined.

If an action has to be carried out, you should state who is going to carry out it out and when.

Example 1

Example of a potentially inadequate communication:

> **DATA**
> Mrs Edwards has a creatinine of 250 …

To which the reply might be 'So what!'

Better practice:

NEED	**DATA**	**ACTION**
Dr Ahmed needs to be told if Mrs Edwards increases above a creatinine of 200	Her creatinine is now 250	Please tell him, I think she may need a nephrostomy

To complete the communication the receiver should say

> **'READ BACK'**
> I will tell Dr Ahmed that Mrs Edwards creatinine is now 250 and that you suggest a nephrostomy

The second communication, including the 'read back' contains seven times more words than the first, and would take about 15 seconds in total to utter it. This is obviously a considerable increase in the time used but it does create a complete and effective communication.

Dr Ahmed might have otherwise spent several minutes tracking down Mrs Edward's creatinine results later in the day, by which time it may be more difficult to arrange the timely insertion of a nephrostomy tube. Thus taking a few seconds more to create a properly structured message might save much more time later.

Example 2

> **DATA**
> 'Mr Bryan's CT head scan is normal'

This might lead someone to think that Mr Bryan is OK and no further treatment is required.

Better practice

NEED	DATA	ACTION
We need to reassess Mr Bryan	His CT head scan is normal	We must consider a lumbar puncture to exclude a subarachnoid haemorrhage

To complete the communication the receiver should say

> **'READ BACK'**
> OK I will arrange a lumbar puncture for Mr Bryan to see if he is has a subarachnoid haemorrhage

Written communication/documentation communication failures

In many ways written communication and documentation failures in healthcare have similar characteristics to verbal communication failures. They also reflect general problems in the way healthcare is organized.

The Frenchay Hospital communications behaviours study[8] noted 'a tendency to seek information from colleagues in preference to printed materials'. The study found that there was poor provision of instructions to locate individuals with whom they might be expected to need to contact.

In one case at Frenchay a junior doctor, new to the department, was asked to arrange an X-ray for a patient. He had not been provided with any relevant documentation to help him. He found a copy of the hospital's internal telephone directory and started to ring numbers in the X-ray department. He made eight telephone calls (of which three were not answered) in order to locate the right person. This process took nearly an hour and four other healthcare professionals were unnecessarily interrupted in their work. A simple departmental handbook with useful contact numbers and other data would save much more time than it would cost to produce.

While one function of written notes is to document the process of care, another equally important one is to provide a channel of communication between staff. With this in mind, it stands to reason that handwriting should be clear, easy to read, and relevant to the situation at hand. The patient's name, record number, and date of birth should be clearly written on each sheet of the clinical note paper. The names and grades of the attending doctors should be noted. Make life easy for people who might feel the need to contact you by noting your bleep number or mobile phone number, so that there is no need to contact the switchboard to find out your number. It is better to make yourself more accessible rather than more inaccessible. The few inappropriate calls you might receive are likely to be more than compensated for by those that are appropriate. Your accessibility may prevent an error from occurring, and if nothing else will earn you a reputation as someone who is easy to contact.

As it is likely that in any week you will make many entries in many patient's notes, get a self-inking rubber stamp with your name and contact number made. At the end of any note you make, stamp your name and number. This can save a not inconsiderable amount of time and effort.

The temporary unavailability of a patient's notes may have been contributory factor in some adverse events. In the context of emergency admissions the patient's notes are not always immediately available. Accepting that this is an inherent failing of a paper-based system of note-keeping (as opposed to an electronic system), try to have as much information available in order to allow you to make safe decisions regarding a patient's care.

Other dangers arise from multiple sets of notes for a single patient. Older patients or those with complex medical problems will often have more than one set of notes. It is important to appreciate that some sets may run concurrently (there may be two sets covering a similar time frame) and not infrequently there is *no* indication in one of these sets of notes that the other set exists. Data, pages of notes, operative records, and correspondence relevant to one admission may be filed in either set! Thus, important information may be fragmented.

The development of electronic patient records should overcome this problem, but until such time as the electronic chart record (ECR) is available for all patients, and while we continue to rely on paper records, remember that there may be more than one set of notes.

References

1 Parker J, Coiera E. Improving clinical communication: a view from psychology. *J Am Med Informatics Assoc* 2000; **7**: 453–61.

2 Joint Commission on Accreditation of Healthcare Organisations (JCAHO). *Sentinel Event Statistics.* 2004.

3 Lingard L, Espin S, Whyte S, *et al.* Communication failures in the operating room: an observational classification of recurrent types and effects. *Qual Saf Health Care* 2004; **13**: 330–4.

4 Barenfanger J, Sautter RL, Lang DL, *et al.* Improving patient safety by repeating (Read-back) telephone reports of critical information. *Am J Clin Pathol* 2004; **121**: 801–3.

5 Grayson R, Billings C. *Information transfer between air traffic control and aircraft: communication problems in flight operations.* NASA Technical Paper 1875. 1981.

6 Report prepared for the Rail Safety and Standards Board London 2006: T365: Collecting and analysing railway safety critical communication error data http://www.rssb.co.uk/Proj_popup.asp?TNumber=365andParent=81andOrd=/.

7 *The Times* newspaper 19 April 2001.

8 **Coiera E, Tombs V.** Communication behaviours in a hospital setting. *Br Med J* 1998; **316**: 673–6.

9 **Holt L.** *'Red for danger'— a history of railway accidents and railway safety precautions.* Bodley Head; 1955.

10 **Little AD.** *Telecommunications: Can it help solve America's healthcare problems?* Cambridge, MA: Arthur D. Little; 1992.

11 **Lowe E.** *Lead responsibility—The facts.* Briefing Paper for Network Rail, September 2003.

12 The Allina Hospital Group's 'alert' phrase is described at www.coloradopatientsafety.org/6-Leonard.ppt/.

13 National Coordinating Council for Medication Error Reporting and Prevention (NCC MERP), http://www.nccmerp.org/.

14 BMA, Junior Doctors Committee, National Patient Safety Agency, NHS Modernisation Agency. *Safe handover: safe patients. Guidance on clinical handover for clinicians and managers.* London: BMA; 2005

15 **Bhabra G, Mackeith S, Monteiro P, Pothier DD.** An experimental comparison of handover methods. *Ann R Coll Surg Engl* 2007; **89**: 298–300.

16 **Makary MA, Mukherjee A, Sexton JB, *et al.*** Operating room briefings and wrong-site surgery. *J Am Coll Surg* 2007; **204**: 236–43.

17 **Leonard M, Graham S, Bonacum D.** The human factor: the critical importance of effective teamwork and communication in providing safe care. *Qual Saf Health Care* 2004; **13**: 185–90.

18 **Sharpe R.** *Assert yourself.* London: Kogan Page Ltd; 1989.

Further reading

Harrison M, Eardley W, McKenna B. Time to hand over our old way of working? *Hosp Med* 2005; **66**: 399–400.

McL Wilson R, Runciman WB, Gibberd RW *et al.* The Quality on Australian Healthcare Study. *Med J Aust* 1995; **163**: 458–71.

Roughton VJ, Severs MP. The junior doctor handover: current practices and future expectations. *J R Coll Physicians Lond* 1996; **30**: 213–14.

Chapter 7

Situation awareness

Most adverse events in healthcare are the result of errors that are made because at least one person is *unaware* of something. A doctor who is unaware of something can be said to have lost so-called **situation awareness**. Situation awareness can therefore be defined very simply as 'knowing what is going on'.

- The surgeon carrying out the right nephrectomy was *unaware* that the tumour was really in the left kidney.
- The consultant was *unaware* that the house officer had not sent the patient's urine for culture.
- The doctor was *unaware* that the poor urine output he was observing in the patient was a symptom of a perforated bladder.
- The doctor was *unaware* that the CT scan had already been carried out and was normal.
- The consultant was *unaware* that the SHO had been given a syringe of vincristine.
- The anaesthetist was *unaware* that the patient's hypoxia was actually caused by a plug of mucus in the ET tube.

And so on ...

In safety-critical industries many accidents have been attributed to **'loss of situation awareness'**. As a result in many safety-critical industries significant resources have been directed to the following reciprocal goals:

- Avoiding the loss of situation awareness during safety-critical operations
- Ensuring good situation awareness during safety-critical operations

---

'Situation awareness' is now an essential concept in human factors science where the complexity of a situation may exceed the ability of the human decision-maker to remain safely in control.

Having complete, accurate, and up-to-the-minute situation awareness is considered to be essential for those who are in control of complex, dynamic systems, and high-risk situations, such as pilots, air traffic controllers, train drivers, railway controllers, engineers in the nuclear and petrochemical industries, military commanders, etc.

Systematic protocols can ensure that front-line healthcare staff are able to achieve high situation awareness in their work.

Situation awareness: definitions

The most authoritative and widely used formal definition of situation awareness is that of the human factors researcher Mica Endsley:[1–3] 'Situation awareness is the perception of elements in the environment within a volume of time and space, the comprehension of their meaning, and the projection of their status in the near future.' The key elements to situation awareness are, therefore, *perception*, *comprehension*, and *projection* of elements in any given situation.

Less formal but more expressive definitions of situation awareness include:

knowing what is going on so you can figure out what to do.[4]

what you need to know not to be surprised.[5]

a shorthand description for keeping track of what is going on around you in a complex, dynamic environment.[6]

Mental models

Limitations in memory and mental processing capabilities mean that humans cannot handle all of the information available to them in their environment. Worse still, when a safety-critical procedure is in progress, a person who is required to make decisions may be unable to directly and immediately perceive all of the critical developments or changes to the system he is attempting to control. Thus, humans have to generate mental representations of operational situations in order to guide their behaviour and decision-making.[7]

In the terminology of cognitive psychology, situation awareness refers to the active content of a decision-maker's mental model or schema of what is currently going on—literally his knowledge of what is going on.

The mental model we have of any given situation is referred to in order to make prompt and appropriate decisions and thus effective actions. Creating and maintaining the correct mental model requires the acquisition, representation, interpretation, and utilization of all relevant information in order to make sense of current events, anticipate future developments, make intelligent decisions and stay in control.

Three levels of situation awareness

Mica Endsley[1,2,3] has identified three levels of situation awareness: perception, comprehension, and projection.

Level 1: situation awareness—perception

This level involves monitoring, cue detection, and simple recognition to produce the most basic level of situation awareness. This is the perception of multiple situational elements (objects, events, people, systems, environmental factors) and their current states (locations, conditions, modes, actions).

Level 2: situation awareness—comprehension

Comprehension involves pattern recognition, interpretation, and evaluation to understand the overall meaning of the perceived elements—how they fit together as a whole, what kind of situation it is, what it means in terms of one's mission goals.

Level 3: situation awareness—projection

The final level of situation awareness involves the mental simulation of the operational situation to determine its possible or probable future state.

Catastrophic loss of situation awareness and the associated syndrome: 'mind lock'

Sometimes it is easier to understand how a particular system works when one element stops working—the function of the failed element is much more obvious than when everything is working smoothly.

In this section we will take a look at some case studies where there was a catastrophic loss of situation awareness and we suggest some psychological processes that may have contributed to the event.

From time to time a frightening event happens in many safety-critical situations and we see examples of this in healthcare:

An operational crisis develops

The operator looks at the available data but makes an incorrect mental model of the situation

The operator then carries out a sequence of actions to remedy the situation, based on the flawed mental model

These actions fail to resolve the crisis and may actually make things worse

$\downarrow$

The operator then becomes overstressed by the developing crisis, resulting in cognitive impairment. This seems to reduce the operator's ability to perceive data that reflects the correct mental model

Crucially, the increased stress levels prevent the operator from recognizing that his actions are actually making the situation worse

$\downarrow$

The time available to resolve the crisis without harm occurring runs out

Three cases studies illustrate this type of scenario:

- the Three Mile Island nuclear power station emergency, 1979
- the Nairobi Boeing 747 'near miss', 1974
- an anaesthetic adverse event.

The Three Mile Island nuclear power station emergency, 1979

The textbook example of this type of loss of situation awareness occurred early on the morning of 27 March 1979 at reactor 2 of the Three Mile Island nuclear power station in Pennsylvania.

At about 4 a.m. a maintenance worker connected a water hose to the wrong valve. This action instantly precipitated a major crisis within the reactor's cooling system.

There were loud bangs throughout the plant as pneumatic valves slammed shut. In the control room alarm bells rang and warning lights flashed. Staff looked around their instrument display to try to understand what was going on. The subsequent investigation revealed that there were serious inadequacies in the way the instrument panel presented vital data.

It is believed that the instruments that the control room staff happened to look at first suggested to them that reactor's cooling system was in a closed condition. Unfortunately, this was the wrong mental model: the system was actually in an open condition.

For the next 2 hours staff tried a series of actions based on the wrong mental model. As a result cooling water was actually being diverted *away* from the overheating reactor core making the crisis even worse.

Fortunately at 6 a.m. the day shift supervisor arrived. He looked at the control panel and instantly made the correct mental model. The correct remedial actions were carried out and the crisis was brought under control.

The Nairobi Boeing 747 Incident, 1974

A similar example of loss of situation awareness very nearly caused a major accident to a British Airways Boeing 747 in September 1974 at Nairobi. This incident was widely discussed in the aviation community at the time and since.

Most of the world's major international airports are built on ground that lies close to sea level. Nairobi is an exception to this as it is located on the East African plateau at an elevation of nearly 5500 feet above sea level.

Unfortunately, the captain failed to remind himself and his colleagues of the high elevation of Nairobi during his 'approach and landing' briefing. In a second error the pilots then misheard an instruction from air traffic control. As a result they thought that they had been cleared to descend to an altitude of 5000 feet (above sea level). This would have been a normal altitude from which to commence the final approach to most of the world's airports. However, at Nairobi the altitude of '5000 feet' is actually below ground level.

The captain programmed the autopilot to descend the aircraft to 5000 feet. When an aircraft is descending at the correct angle towards the runway, two of the cockpit instruments show a 'centred' indication (neither too high nor too low). However, the captain noticed that these instruments were showing that the aircraft was not at the correct angle. There was thick cloud in the area and it was not possible to determine the aircraft's position visually.

In such a situation there are two possible mental models that can be made: theory A, the aircraft is too high and is above the correct angle, and theory B, the aircraft is too low and below the correct angle.

The captain seems to have adopted theory A and adjusted the autopilot to increase the aircraft's angle of descent. In fact the aircraft was already too low and the captain's action made the situation worse. The flight engineer looked at the instruments and recognized that the captain's actions were not causing the instrument indications to move toward the centre. Unfortunately, the captain cut him short before he could develop his thoughts and give the captain a structured comment on the situation and point to the critical anomalous instrument indications.

For 2 minutes or so the captain's mind remained locked on the idea that they were too high and he failed to recognize the fact that his actions were not correcting the problem. The aircraft was now in a precarious position, less than a minute from hitting the ground. The aircraft's warning systems then started to warn the crew of the rapid closure rate with the ground with an automated voice calling out, 'PULL UP, PULL UP,

PULL UP'. Other warnings pointed out the excessive displacement below the correct angle.

These warnings were not consistent with the captain's mental model that he was too high and so he ignored them.

At the very last moment the aircraft descended out of the clouds and the captain saw the treetops ahead. He managed to arrest the descent and climb the aircraft away to make a second, successful approach. The aircraft had come within 70 feet of the ground.

Hypoxic cardiac arrest following ventilator disconnection

During an operation,[8] a patient became disconnected from the ventilator and consequently suffered a hypoxic cardiac arrest. The disconnection was not noticed at the time by the anaesthetist. The hypoxia initially caused increases in the heart rate and blood pressure, which the anaesthetist interpreted as indicating inadequate anaesthesia.

He increased the inspired concentration of anaesthetic agent and administered an intravenous beta blocker. He attributed the subsequent decreases in the heart rate and blood pressure and the cardiac arrest to the beta blocker.

In spite of a number of indications to the contrary over several minutes his mental model throughout was that there was inadequate anaesthesia. As a result of this event the patient was left in a persistent vegetative state.

It is important that healthcare professionals understand the psychology behind flawed mental modelling. Use of the appropriate terminology when they discuss the problem with colleagues would be helpful in reducing the ramifications of loss of situation awareness. If appropriate terminology is not used it is difficult to prevent a crude blame culture.

Experience in all safety-critical industries shows that even the most experienced and conscientious professionals, with previously blameless careers, can fall victim to a flawed mental model and ignore all of the consequent 'red flags'.

The answer is to arrange training sessions for simulated emergencies. When a confusing crisis develops, the team leader should actively seek input from other team members.

An aviation training film of one such simulated emergency in an aircraft simulator shows a confused captain asking his crew:

> Can any one think of anything that we need to do that we have not done?

Fortunately, in the scenario reconstructed for the training film, the flight engineer did have an idea that helped to resolve the crisis.

As a senior surgeon or physician in a crisis, ask your team (junior doctors, nurses, the anaesthetist) to help you out—they might have spotted an obvious cause for the problem that you may not have noticed.

Understanding loss of situation awareness

Situation awareness can be lost as a result of three types of problems.

1. Problems with the data. **Data problems** might be caused by situations such as:
   - incomplete or incorrect data being used to create the mental model (e.g. missing information in the patient's notes)
   - procedures to prepare or handle data are inadequate or not followed properly (e.g. absence of formal checking procedures).

2. **Processing problems**:
   - cognitive failures where the data are processed into an erroneous mental model. This might be because one set of data is assessed incorrectly as being more reliable than other data.

3. **Catalyst events**, which might include:
   - events that persuade the subject that certain valid data is invalid or vice versa
   - a deceptive situation arises (e.g. two patients with similar names arrive in the department at the same time or a patient responds abnormally to a treatment).

Standard procedures, checklists, and pre-operative briefings can be used to address data problems.

High reliability organizations appreciate that professionals working in safety-critical environments must have some understanding of how problems of cognition arise in order to prevent such problems arising or in order to deal with the consequences of such a situation when it occurs.

Cognitive failures: the role of mental models/the psychology of mistakes

We cannot possibly be conscious of every detail of a given situation that is going on around us. If we were, our minds would be so full of irrelevant details that we would be quite unable to think.

Mental models are necessary to allow the brain, with its limited data processing capacity, but high cognitive ability, to deal efficiently with the torrent of stimuli.

A good example of a mental model that each of us use on a daily basis is the mental model of our journey to and from work. We have such an effective mental model of the route to and from work that we can drive home from work while thinking about a particular problem that we have encountered during the day. When we get home we might realize that we have only a vague recollection of parts of the journey. Effectively we drove home 'on autopilot' with the brain running a series of complex skill-based programmes (operating the car, changing a CD in the CD player and selecting a song, finding the route home, taking a phone call, avoiding collisions with other road users) without any conscious effort at all.

The price we pay for such 'virtuosity' is the possibility of bias, oversight, or distortion in our perception of the data.

The brain processes this torrent of stimulation through a *single channel* system. In other words, it can only do one piece of processing at a time. The only way that all of this huge sensory input can be handled is by a process called 'schematic processing'.

The mind searches for similarities between the situation being sensed and a previously experienced situation or schema (scheme of things). If a 'fit' is found all incoming data are processed in accordance with the selected schema, the assumed model.

Only the very small amount of information/sensations that are required to control the situation is sought. Other input, which does not seem critical or relevant to the situation, is filtered out. Only those sensations that are required to operate effectively are passed on. One can also think of this being a mental template. Sensations or stimuli lying outside the template are cut-off. We also filter out undesired sensations. If you are in a room with loud air conditioning noise, we are able to subconsciously delete the noise.

The problem is that these 'filtering' functions can occasionally filter out important data that you need to carry out your work safely. You will not be aware that this is happening. The brain is able to handle the smaller volume of sensory input that emerges once irrelevant information has been screened out. As no processing or screening can be done until a schema is adopted there is a strong need to find a schema quickly.

Mental models: the problems

One problem with mental models is that occasionally false ones can be adopted and can then be very difficult to dislodge. In healthcare this is manifest when a wrong diagnosis is made and the diagnosis is not modified when evidence arises suggesting the original diagnosis might not be correct. The following psychological processes can induce this flawed mental modelling.

Primacy effect

The primacy effect describes our tendency to take the first hypothesis for which two or more pieces of confirmatory evidence appear.[9]

When our primeval ancestors met another human being it was important to establish if he were friend or foe very quickly. The world would thus comprise good people or bad people.

Read the following text about the activities of a student called Jim.

Jim left the house to get some stationery. He walked out into the sun-filled street with two of his friends, basking in the sun as he walked. Jim entered the stationery shop, which was full of people. Jim joked with a friend while he waited to catch the assistant's eye. On his way out, he stopped to chat with a school friend who was just coming into the shop. Leaving the shop, he walked toward the school. On his way he met the girl to whom he had been introduced the night before. They talked for a short while, and then Jim turned for school. After school, Jim left the classroom alone. Leaving the school, he started on his long walk home. The street was brilliantly filled with sunshine but Jim walked down the street on the shady side. Coming down the street toward him, he saw in the distance the pretty girl whom he had met on the previous evening. Jim immediately crossed the street and entered a bar. The bar was crowded with students, and he noticed a few familiar faces. Jim waited quietly until he caught the barman's eye and then gave his order. Taking his drink, he sat down at a side table. When he had finished his drink he went home.

Adapted from Luchins[10]

Seventy-eight per cent of people who read this description of Jim's activities assessed him as 'friendly'.[10]

This account was then re-written so that it begins with the second half of the text first and the first half second (beginning 'After school, Jim left'). This version was shown to a second group of subjects. The result was very different and only 19% found him 'friendly'.

The two halves of the piece appear to contain very different behaviours. In the first half he appears to be very sociable, in the second half he seems to avoid social contact.

As both groups of subjects have exactly the same information it seems that, in general, the first information we receive has the greater impact on our over-all impressions. This is known as the primacy effect.

When we are first attempting to form our impressions of a person, we actively search in memory for the person model (also called a stereotype) that best matches the incoming data. Reasonably quickly, we make a preliminary decision: this person is friendly (or some such judgement).

As we then assimilate any further information we dismiss any discrepant information as not consistent with the adopted mental model. For example, when explicitly asked to account for the apparent contradictions in Jim's behaviour, subjects sometimes say that Jim is really friendly but was probably tired by the end of the day.[10] Our theory about Jim, which has already been established, shapes our perception of all subsequent data about him.

In a healthcare setting when we meet a new colleague for the first time we are more likely to attempt to make an assessment about his competence rather than his friendliness.

The primacy effect is not only evident when assessing people, it is also present when assessing situations; for example, diagnosing a patient's condition. In accident and emergency medicine, a dangerous example of the primacy effect is the assumption that someone who 'smells of alcohol' and has a reduced conscious level is suffering from alcohol intoxication. In fact the actual cause of confusion may be hypoglycaemia or a concealed head injury.

The primacy effect seems to have influenced the adoption of the wrong mental model by the supervisor in the control room at Three Mile Island and the captain of the Boeing 737 involved in the 1989 Kegworth accident, where the healthy engine was shut down rather than the engine that was on fire.

Having accepted the wrong mental model possibly as a result of the primacy effect, the mind then seeks evidence to support the first (flawed) assumption, while indications confirming a second (correct) assumption are subcon-sciously rejected. This is called 'confirmation bias'.

Confirmation bias

> The human mind when it has once adopted an opinion draws all things else to support and agree with it
>
> Sir Francis Bacon (1620)

Sir Francis Bacon clearly understood the existence of the phenomenon that we nowadays call confirmation bias. Confirmation bias is an unconscious prefer-ence for evidence that fits, confirms, or supports our beliefs in preference to evidence that opposes our beliefs.

In attempting to save cognitive effort we do not so much search out confirmatory evidence so much as to wait for consistent data to come along. It seems that contradictory evidence is 'screened out' without our being aware of it.

Thus operators are more likely to reject any information that is not consistent with their expectations, rather than update their mental model. The latter has a cost that operators cannot always afford in time-critical situations. In the end, data can be reinterpreted to fit the model that operators have of a situation.[6] This confirmation bias is probably the outcome of an economy-driven reasoning: following a line of least effort,[11] operators can treat random data as meaningful if it matches their vision of the world.

In a 'mind-lock' crisis situation, operators erroneously maintain as valid a mental model that ought to be obvious to them is completely flawed.

We may even rate evidence that is actually neutral as supporting evidence. In other words we interpret the 'evidence' in a way that supports our views. The study below is an example of how subjects on both sides of an issue respectively rated neutral evidence as supporting their views.

Allan Mazur[12] conducted a survey to determine how the 1979 Three Mile Island nuclear power station incident affected the opinions of 42 scientists on the subject of nuclear power development. All of the scientists had previously made their views known. *Despite the events that took place at Three Mile Island, none of the scientists had changed their views.* Instead, most of them took the near-accident as being evidence for whichever view they held in the first place. Proponents of nuclear power development saw the incident as evidence that safety systems in nuclear power plants work, reinforcing their initial view that such plants are safe. At the same time, opponents of nuclear power development saw the incident as a serious adverse event that was averted by the narrowest of margins, and so was evidence that nuclear power plants are dangerous and should be opposed. The same 'evidence', therefore, was used as evidence for a claim and as evidence against it!

Subconscious 'fabrication' of data

In situations where there is a break in the flow of data it seems that we have a strong tendency to 'make up' data to fill in the gap. We also create data to enable us to link pieces of information. Psychologists call these fabricated elements **'Inferences'**.

- ◆ Emily saw the ice cream van
- ◆ She remembered the pocket money
- ◆ She rushed into the house

It is almost impossible to read those 16 words without imagining the scene and assuming that the child has rushed inside to get money to buy an ice cream. We may even visualize a particular local street where we have seen an ice cream van selling ice cream to children. We have made inferences based on our schema of children's behaviour when ice cream vans appear. These 'inferences' may be false and lure us into creating the wrong schema.

We are likely to *infer* that Emily is a child, that she likes ice cream and that she has gone home to get money for the ice cream. When asked whether the ice cream van was stationary or approaching Emily when she saw it, most people would say that it could not have already passed her by, otherwise there would have been no point in Emily's rushing into the house to get the money.

Wherever there is an apparent interruption in the flow of sensation the subconscious will tend to fill in gaps in order to complete the picture. We will not be aware of this 'fabrication' and we believe we have actually perceived the fabricated elements.

Assumed connection

We have a strong tendency to assume that some of the events going on around us are linked by a single common factor. This problem, if unchecked, can lead to people believing in conspiracy theories and, in extremis, paranoia.

The failure of the supervisor in the Three Mile Island Nuclear power plant incident to abandon his flawed mental model was partly due to his confusion about the cause of the problems he was having with the emergency feed water-cooling system. He assumed that the latter problems were connected with initial failure. In fact they were completely unconnected. (His technical training had emphasized that the emergency feed water cooling system was completely independent of the plant's main cooling system.) Unfortunately, he wasted his mental resources trying to fathom the connection.

The problem is that the 'assumed connection' thought process leads to unnecessary mental effort being applied to finding the common factor that has supposedly instigated both events.

We become intrigued by the mental challenge of solving the mystery. While we are considering the mystery, we may miss some development to which we really ought to attend. This distraction can lead to serious errors.

A patient developed difficulty breathing following an appendicectomy. It was initially thought this was due to abdominal pain restricting diaphragmatic movement. For several days this remained the diagnosis. The difficulty breathing persisted. It was later discovered that the patient had developed a spontaneous pneumothorax.

Unreliable evidence

It seems that sometimes we can continue to believe something even when we know that the reason for believing it in the first place is unreliable or even completely untrue.

A group of subjects was shown a seemingly authentic 'research paper' that contained convincing evidence that fire fighters had attitudes that made them more likely to take life-threatening risks.[13] Another group was presented with another paper showing the opposite conclusion.

Later both groups were told that the papers were based on totally fictitious evidence. Despite this, when the two groups were subsequently asked to list people in occupations who were likely to take risks or avoid risks, the people in each group ranked fire fighters on the basis of what they had read in the 'research' paper. They did this even though they knew that the evidence that they were basing their rankings on was completely untrue.

Thus the psychological processes referred to above can adversely affect how we process and analyse data to create mental models.

Ensuring high situation awareness

High reliability organizations give a great deal of thought to ensuring that their personnel achieve high situation awareness in safety-critical situations. This is achieved by:

- Using standard operating procedures (SOPs), checklists, briefings, and announcements.
- Making documentation, equipment displays, etc. as clear as possible.
- Creating 'team situation awareness'.

One important aspect of SOPs is that they create expectations. As a result when an unexpected event occurs it is more likely to be drawn to the attention of team members promptly. This may well be before a flawed mental model is adopted or other coincidental events cause further confusion.

Checklists and checking procedures: as tools to enhance situation awareness

The first 8 case studies in Chapter 4 could have been prevented had the checking procedures worked effectively. Seven of the patients involved died as a direct result of a failure of the checking process.

While clinicians are required to carry out checks to confirm patient identity or that the correct procedure is to be carried out or the correct drug is given, the system fails to produce adequate reliability. This is because the system does not specify in detail exactly:

- how a check is to be carried out
- when a check is to be carried out
- who is to carry out a check.

Checks in healthcare are often carried out in silence and it is assumed that if no one says anything to the contrary that the checks have revealed nothing amiss. It was exactly this assumption that led to the 'Herald of Free Enterprise' disaster where a cross-channel ferry capsized within minutes of leaving harbour because no one had checked that the bow doors, through which vehicles were loaded, were closed. They were in fact open! Official Townsend Thorensen Shipping Company procedures allowed the captain to assume that the ship's bow doors were closed unless someone told him that they were not. Thus the captain received the same input when the doors were closed as when the check had not been carried out at all. Such an ambiguity is not tolerated in high reliability organizations.

Checklists

A checklist is an algorithmic listing of actions to be performed when carrying out a complex procedure when in a safety-critical environment. Checklists are used extensively in high reliability organizations. Personnel receive detailed training in precisely how to carry out the checklist and there are regular audits on compliance.

Introduction of checklists—and what can happen when checklists are not used The prerequisite for the successful introduction of a checklist is a receptive 'attitude' on the part of the operators. Receptivity is, in turn, strongly influenced by the support and commitment of senior personnel and management.

In 1983 the Federal Aviation Agency (FAA), the civil aviation regulatory authority in America, sent its Operations Inspectors to observe airline crews using the 'Before-take-off-checklist'.[14] They found that pilots in most of the airlines carried out the checklists with the required level of diligence; however, in two major airlines, there was serious cause for concern. The inspectors' report into these airlines mentioned 'inadequate standards, breaches of regulations, flagrant disregard of cockpit discipline and checklists done from memory'. Analysis of incident and accident records revealed that these airlines also suffered more than their fair share of such events.

The FAA wrote to these airlines to express their concerns. Both airlines rejected the criticism and made no proposals to change their training. They said their pilots' performance was acceptable.

Fate punished the airlines cruelly for their complacent attitude. On 16 August 1987 flight 255 failed to climb after take-off from Detroit, struck buildings beyond the runway and exploded in a horrific fireball—156 people perished. Investigations revealed that the pilots had not set the flaps correctly for take-off and the cockpit voice recording showed that they had not used the 'before-take-off-checklist'. One might have imagined that other pilots would learn the obvious lesson. Alas they did not.

On 31 August 1988 flight 1141 crashed on take-off from Dallas in almost identical circumstances. Fortunately, no buildings stood on the ground beyond the runway at Dallas and only 14 people died in the accident. Chillingly, the cockpit voice recording revealed exactly the same lack of discipline in the cockpit before take-off.

A video reconstruction was made of the Detroit accident using computer-generated imagery. It is still used on training courses to demonstrate the terrible consequences of laxity in the use of checklists.

As a result of the Detroit and Dallas accidents, the FAA carried out more intensive operational standards observations and ensured that airlines took immediate measures to address any shortcomings.

In the past, safety-critical industries issued checklists to their staff but gave little or no guidance as to how to use them. This is still the case in healthcare. High reliability organizations now appreciate that it is necessary to give very precise instructions to their personnel on how to use the checklist. The exact words to be used are sometimes specified.

An important element in checklist procedures is **'pointing and calling'**. This is where the team member points to the instrument display, the control lever or the words in the document to be checked and calls out what he sees. Contrary to what your mother told you, this is *not* rude!

Wherever possible two people should be involved in carrying out the checklist. One person, usually the junior, reads out the item to be checked and the other responds, physically pointing to the item. The reader ensures that all the items are checked.

Types of checklist There are two types of checklist:

1. **'Read and do checklist'.** This is used when a team face an abnormal or a crisis situation, and a specific checklist is used to remind them of the actions to be carried out and the appropriate, correct, and safe sequence in which to carry them out.

   A 'Read and do Checklist' can also be used to help with the correct diagnosis of the underlying problem that requires the use of the checklist. These checks can be sequenced to eliminate the most likely possible diagnoses first.

   The stress of the situation may otherwise cause the team to overlook important elements, steps, or diagnoses.

2. **'Challenge and response' checklist.** This is used in more routine situations to confirm that all the necessary preparatory actions have already been carried out before a procedure commences.

Table 7.1 shows part of the pre-anaesthesia checklist as used in the University Hospital, Leiden, in the Netherlands. The complete checking process includes drugs, intubation materials, and the patient.

Table 7.1 The pre-anaesthesia checklist used in the University Hospital, Leiden, the Netherlands

Anaesthetist 1: Challenge	Anaesthetist 2: Response
'Check electrical connections'	'Electricals OK'
'Check alarm limits'	'Alarm OK'
'Check gas connections'	'Gas OK'
'Check and set O_2 meter'	'Oxymeter OK'
'Check spriolog calibration'	'Spriolog Calibrated'
'Check gas flow'	'Flows OK'
'Check vapourizer'	'Vapourizer OK'
'Check suction'	'Suction OK'
'Check circle system'	'Circle OK'
'Check O_2 bypass'	'Bypass OK'
'Leakage test'	'Test OK'
'Check function control IPPV'	'IPPV OK'
'Check and set volume connections'	'Volume OK and set'
'Check and set frequency'	'Frequency OK and set'
'Check and set PEEP'	'PEEP OK and set'
'Check and set trigger'	'Trigger OK and set'
'Set selector IPPV/ SPONT/ MAN'	'Selector Set for ... '
'Set selector O_2/N_2O/O_2 AIR'	'Selector Set for ... '

Briefings and announcements: as tools to enhance situation awareness

Briefings, although standard practice in 'high-risk' industries, the military, and the police, are uncommon in healthcare. All too often there is evidence that in adverse events individual members of a team of doctors and nurses (in an operating theatre, for example) had divergent expectations of what they thought was going to happen.

Progressive healthcare organizations in North America now formally require briefings for obstetric, rapid response, ICU, and other teams.

The following briefing guide has been developed by surgical teams at the Orange County, Los Angeles hospital of the Kaiser Permanente group in the United States.[15] It has now been formally adopted into their care processes.

The briefing categories are broken into four sections. The surgical category begins with the surgeon telling other team members what he/she thinks they needed to know in a given case. It is then everyone else's turn to tell the surgeon what they need to know. For example, the operating room nurses want to know if the surgeon is on call, because they will have to answer the surgeon's pager frequently during the case. During the development of the briefing system surgeons were surprised to learn how much impact this would have on the nurses during the surgery. The development of the briefing procedure has allowed people who had worked together for years to discover basic insights into how their behaviour or transfer of information affects others.

The pre-surgery briefing chart shown in Fig. 7.1 is the third version developed by the team. It is a template showing the potential topics for the surgical team to cover, which they use as relevant to the case at hand. The briefing is done only after the patient is anaesthetized, that being the only time all members of the team are physically present together.

As an alternative, other healthcare organizations, believing that it is preferable to brief prior to the induction of anaesthesia, have chosen to brief in the operating room with the patient awake. The initial concern that briefing with the patient might infer from this that the team did not know what they were doing has not been borne out; early indications are that patients really like the process. It is presented to the patient as a last opportunity for the surgical team to make sure they are all 'on the same page' and doing everything correctly.

Thus, a surgeon should carry out a briefing describing the expected course of events and any special features of a procedure. This is particularly important when the procedure is rarely performed, where there are abnormal conditions

Surgeon	Circulator	Scrub	Anesthesia
• ID patient and site • What type of surgery? • Realistic time estimate • What is the desired position? • Any special equipment needed? • Is this a standard procedure or are there special needs? • Are there any anticipated problems? • Will we need pathology? • Is a radiology C-arm or portable X-ray requested, and will it be needed? • Are there any special intraoperative requests, i.e., wake-up, and hypothermia? • Plan to transfuse? "Wet versus dry" • Use of drugs on the field? • Do you want lines? • Postop pain management-special request (CLE, blocks, etc.)	• Identify patient site and marking • Allergies? • Verification of medication on the back table • X-ray available and other special services, (i.e., x-rays, pacemaker, cell saver, sales rep, laser) • Blood available?	• Do we have all the instruments? • Are there any instruments missing from the tray? • Are all the instruments working? • What special instrumentation do we need? • Do they have a question about the instruments?	• What type of anesthesia will be used? • Risks? • Should we anticipate any problems? • Any special needs – positioning, medications? • Special lines driven by anesthesia

Fig. 7.1 Pre-surgery briefing chart.

or when a new member has joined the surgical team. In the latter case it might be helpful to allocate responsibilities. Anecdotal evidence suggests such responsibilities are not always adequately defined.

Mention might be made of potential error-inducing situations. So, for example, the surgeon might at this juncture remind every member of the team that every patient will need intermittent pneumatic compression boots on and that the each operation should not start until they are applied and are switched on. Where two patients have similar names (ideally best avoided) then the attention of all team members to the requirement for double-checking which patient is being operated on could be made.

It might be useful to announce the approximate duration of the procedure. The author was informed of a case where, at an early stage in a surgical procedure one morning, the surgeon looked at the theatre clock and made a remark to the effect that they would be lucky if they were out of there by lunchtime. This was a surprise for the anaesthetist who had prepared the patient for a much shorter procedure. A discussion ensued that revealed that there were significant differences between the expectations of members of the surgical and anaesthetic team. These differences between the expectations had implications for the anaesthesia and could have produced distracting interactions at a critical point in the procedure.

In order to create a 'risk-conscious' atmosphere, the surgeon might complete his briefing with an invitation as follows:

> If at any point you spot something that you don't think I have noticed, please tell me straight away. If you think I am making a mistake, you might be right!

It often enhances team situation awareness if the steps of the procedure are announced as they are happening. This might involve announcing events or actions that might be obvious.

Human factors experts working for the railway industry have been considering the problem of how to reduce cases of SPAD, 'signals passed at danger', in other words trains not stopping at red lights. One error management strategy that seems to be promising is 'pointing and calling' railway signals. The train driver points to each signal as he approaches it and calls out loud the colour of the light that it is showing. He does this even though he is alone in his cab. Japanese railways have made this practice mandatory.[16] Human factors experts believe that this verbalization (even simply talking to oneself) raises awareness and seems to transfer the datum from short-term memory into longer-term memory.

Creating team situation awareness: as a tool to enhance situation awareness

During patient safety courses delegates are shown an image that contains a number of objects of different types. They are asked to count how many objects of one type they can see in the image. Afterwards everyone agrees that it is an extremely simple task.

In spite of this it is interesting to note that less than half of the delegates are able to spot all of the objects. When told that there are more objects to spot some people completely refuse to believe that they could have missed any as it seems to be so simple an image. It is only when the delegates are allowed to communicate with each other that the delegates who see all of the objects are able point them all out to the others.

This exercise shows that situation awareness differs markedly between individuals even in extremely straight-forward situations. How much more likely is it, therefore, that it will vary in complex situations?

High reliability organizations have developed a solution to this problem: This is 'team situation awareness'. This is achieved by creating a cultural atmosphere and procedures where all the team members can share their individual situation awareness in order to produce team situation awareness.

Clearly the procedures described above—under 'Briefings and announcements' are able to enhance team situation awareness.

Two special cases involving loss of situation awareness

There are two situations in surgical practice where loss of situation awareness can lead to serious errors and where simple techniques can reduce the likelihood of such errors from occurring:

- ◆ wrong site/wrong side/wrong patient/wrong procedure surgery
- ◆ retained swabs and surgical instruments.

The techniques to reduce the likelihood of these errors from occurring include pre-procedure briefings that involve all members of the operating theatre team and the use of checklists.

Situation awareness: wrong site/wrong side/wrong patient/wrong procedure surgery

Operating on the wrong patient, wrong site or wrong side clearly involves a loss of situation awareness.

> I thought I was operating on Mr Smith, when in reality it was Mr Jones who was on the operating table
>
> I thought it was the right kidney we had to remove—I didn't realise it was really the left kidney

In these two scenarios, the surgeon's mental model of the situation does not match reality. These are not hypothetical cases—remarkable though it may seem, surgeons really do sometimes operate on the wrong patient, or at the wrong site or remove the wrong leg! Not surprisingly, the general public regard such errors as unforgivable and intense media scrutiny of the individual surgeon is common (the initial media 'analysis' always focuses on the individual rather than the system failures!).

Wrong site/wrong side/wrong patient/wrong procedure surgery: What is it?

- ◆ *Wrong site surgery:* the performance of an operation or surgical procedure on the wrong part of the body (surgery at the wrong anatomical site). The commonest type of wrong site surgery is wrong *side* surgery (Tables 7.2 and 7.3).

Table 7.2 Wrong site surgery occurs more frequently than wrong patient and wrong procedure surgery

	%
Wrong part or wrong side surgery	76
Wrong patient	13
Wrong procedure	11

Data from root cause analysis of 126 cases of wrong-site surgery in a JCAHO database.[30]

Table 7.3 From the Pennsylvania Patient Safety Authority[23]

	n (%)
Wrong part or wrong site surgery	358 (83)
Wrong patient	34 (8)
Wrong procedure	39 (9)

Other types of wrong site surgery include—wrong spinal level; correct side but wrong digit; correct side but medial/lateral error; correct side but anterior/posterior error; correct side but proximal/distal error. Most wrong site surgery involves symmetrical anatomic structures.

- *Wrong procedure surgery:* the performance of an operation other than that intended or indicated.
- *Wrong person surgery:* the performance of an operation or procedure on a person other than the one for whom the procedure was intended.

Wrong *side* surgery is the commonest type of wrong site surgery

Wrong site surgery occurs more frequently than wrong patient and wrong procedure surgery (Table 7.2, Table 7.3).

A real-life example: loss of situation awareness leading to a near-miss wrong patient/side operation

This situation occurred recently to one of the authors. A near miss occurred. Fortunately, no harm to any patient was done but one surgeon had a very nasty scare.

I had just finished performing a right ureteroscopic stone fragmentation on a patient, Mr R. Having written the operative note I had taken the patients records down to the recovery room myself. On returning to the operating theatre, my registrar was already scrubbed and ready to perform the next operation—a left ureteroscopy on the next patient, Mr L.

I asked him some detail about Mr L's case and it became apparent that my registrar had not read the patient's notes. 'But I have looked at the X-rays' he said. We both crossed over to the computer screen to look at the digital images. The X-ray images of the previous patient, Mr R (who had just undergone a *RIGHT* ureteroscopy), were still on the screen. No one had uploaded Mr L's digital X-ray images (left ureteroscopy). My registrar obviously thought the X-rays on the screen (Mr R's) were those of the patient on the operating table (Mr L). He clearly also thought the patient on the operating table was Mr R—when of course it was Mr L. He had not checked.

He was, therefore, about to operate on the wrong patient *and* on the wrong side. He had lost (in fact he had never had) situation awareness.

When I pointed this error out to him, the expression on his face changed to an ashen grey colour. He was clearly stunned by what he had been about to do.

Fortunately, no harm had been done to the patient, but this was a very unpleasant experience for my registrar. Thank goodness we hadn't been doing a nephrectomy and that I hadn't left him to his own devices!

The root cause of this near miss

The operating surgeon (the registrar) had not *personally* checked the identity or side of the intended procedure against another item of information such as the notes or the consent form. He had assumed that all of this had been done for him. This is a good example of social shirking—'I thought you'd checked' (this is *exactly* what the registrar in the South Wales wrong kidney case said).

No *cross-check* with another member of staff had been made. Fortunately, as the consultant surgeon in charge of the case I always check the identity of the patient myself, even if my registrar is doing the operation, and I confirm the site and side of the operation and check that antibiotic and deep vein thrombosis prophylaxis has been given. This additional check would have prevented a wrong side procedure in this instance.

We will discuss techniques of prevention of wrong site and wrong side surgery later in this chapter, but in brief as the operating surgeon make sure *you* do the critical safety checks and involve another member of the theatre team, such as the anaesthetist, in the process. Check the patient's identity (cross-check the hospital notes with the identity wrist band), confirm the correct site and side of the operation (and while doing all of this, why not also check that appropriate antibiotic and deep vein thrombosis prophylaxis has been given or applied). If some other individual has already checked all of these items, it doesn't matter. It will take about a minute for you to re-check and you can rest assured that you are playing safe. Do these checks with another member of the theatre team, i.e. *cross*-check.

As the consultant in charge of a case make sure your junior doctors are fully versed in the concept of correct site/side/patient cross-checking. If they are unable to do this very simple check, then it is unlikely that you can trust them to safely perform a more complex procedure, such as an operation. You will need to regularly monitor your junior doctor's performance in this checking process. Tell them that you will do this—not because you don't trust them, but because they are human and like any human (no matter how brilliant, no matter how conscientious) they will, from time to time commit an error. Reverse roles from time to time—ask them to monitor your checking process and to constructively criticize you if you forget to do what you have asked them to do.

An aside. Not knowing your patient is a potent source of error. Turning up to the operating theatre to do an operation on a patient without being familiar with their case is a recipe for disaster. As the consultant in charge of this case, I felt a certain responsibility for what had happened. I had not been forceful enough in ensuring that my residents had acquainted themselves with details of the case. I had not been forceful enough in ensuring that the residents carried out a process of cross-checking with the anaesthetist that they were about to operate on the correct patient, on the correct side and on the correct site. This failure to ensure the residents were knowledgeable in such matters could be called a systems failure.

I now have a rule that I apply to residents who wish to operate on patients under my care. It is called the Kourambas rule after John Kourambas, an Australian Urological Surgeon from Melbourne, who worked in Oxford some years ago. John Kourambas prided himself on the fact that he always knew more about the case than his consultant. The rule is simple. If I know more about the case, I do the operation with the resident as assistant. If the resident passes the Kourambas test they have the opportunity of doing the case, with me as assistant.

I also instruct my residents that failure to cross-check the patient's name and hospital number against the patient's medical records is a reason for them being denied the opportunity to do the operation. Most people are sensible enough to understand the reasons for this rule—after all, how can I trust a surgeon to operate safely if he can't even operate on the correct patient. I make random checks to ensure that correct patient identification is being carried out, not because my residents are wicked, mistrustful people, but because I know they are human and I know that from time to time they make lapses. An important aspect of high reliability organization safety practice (discussed later) is monitoring of staff to ensure maintenance of compliance with safety measures. This is not spying—it's just sensible given the inevitability that humans are error prone.

Ask another member of the team to help you cross-check the identity of the patient, the type of operation and its site and side before you embark on any procedure.

Use several sources of information, such as the patient's identity band, the notes and X-rays, to ensure you both understand the situation.

Ideally, check that the patient is the correct patient *before* they are anaesthetized by asking them to confirm their address to you. Explain to the patient that this is an additional safety check so as not to alarm them.

Another real-life example: loss of situation awareness leading to a wrong patient procedure

It is not just surgeons who perform wrong patient procedures! Other healthcare workers have been known to commit this error.

The following case is a good example of loss of situation awareness, leading to a wrong patient procedure. Joan Morris was admitted to a teaching hospital in the USA for cerebral angiography. She had undergone cerebral angiography and was transferred to the oncology ward rather than to her original bed as there were no beds on the ward she would normally have been sent to. She mistakenly underwent an invasive cardiac electrophysiology study the following morning—a procedure that was intended for another patient called Jane Morrison.

Jane Morrison's delayed cardiac electrophysiology study was scheduled as the first electrophysiology case for the early morning of the day of Joan Morris's planned discharge. The electrophysiology nurse (RN1) telephoned the cardiac ward and asked for 'patient Morrison'. The person answering the telephone incorrectly stated that Jane Morrison had been moved to the oncology ward, when she was, in fact, still on the cardiac ward. It was actually Joan Morris who had been transferred to the oncology ward after her cerebral angiogram. Thus, there was a loss of situation awareness and this was due to absent active identification.

RN1 called the oncology ward, where Joan Morris had been transferred after her cerebral angiography. Joan Morris's nurse, RN2 (who was nearing the end of her shift), agreed to transport Joan for the electrophysiology procedure. Joan Morris stated that she was unaware of plans for an electrophysiology procedure, she did not want to undergo it, and she was feeling nauseated.

Despite these protestations RN2 brought Joan Morris to the electrophysiology laboratory. After the patient again expressed reluctance to undergo the procedure, the electrophysiology nurse, RN1, paged the electrophysiology doctor, who returned the page promptly. He asked to speak with the patient on the telephone. The doctor had briefly met Jane Morrison (the correct patient who was scheduled to the cardiac study) the night before but did not realize he was now speaking to a different patient. Again, there was loss of situation awareness due to absent active identification. The doctor was somewhat surprised to hear of her reluctance to undergo the procedure because she had not expressed this concern the night before. After speaking with Ms Morris, he instructed RN1 to administer an intravenous anti-emetic and stated that the patient had agreed to proceed.

The electrophysiology charge nurse arrived and was told by RN1 that a patient scheduled for an early start had arrived. No patient name was used in this conversation. Once again, there was loss of situation awareness due to absent active identification. The charge nurse checked the electrophysiology schedule and then left to attend to other duties. RN3 placed the patient on the table, attached monitors, and spoke to the patient about her procedure. Joan Morris stated that she had 'fainted,' which seemed to RN3 to be a reasonable indication for an electrophysiology procedure (an incorrect mental model was thus confirmed).

A resident from the neurosurgery team on his morning rounds was surprised to find Joan Morris out of her room. After learning of the electrophysiology procedure, he came down to the electrophysiology laboratory and demanded to know 'why my patient' (not using her name—and so again not actively identifying the patient) was there, as he was unaware of an order for this procedure. RN1 informed the resident that the patient had been bumped twice already but was now being taken as the first case of the day. The resident left the electrophysiology laboratory assuming that his chief had ordered the study without telling him.

An additional electrophysiology nurse (RN4) and the electrophysiology doctor arrived. The doctor stood outside the procedure room at the computer console and could not see the patient's face because her head was draped. The fellow initiated the procedure, inserting a femoral artery sheath and began programmed stimulation of the heart via an intracardiac electrophysiology catheter.

A nurse from the telemetry floor, RN5, telephoned the electrophysiology laboratory to find out why no one had called for Jane Morrison (the correct patient). RN3 took the call and, after consulting with RN4 about the expected completion time for the current case (Joan Morris), advised RN5 to send Jane Morrison down at 10 a.m.

The electrophysiology charge nurse, making patient stickers for the morning cases, noticed that 'Joan Morris' did not match any of the five names listed in the morning log. Entering the electrophysiology laboratory, she questioned the fellow about the patient names. He said, 'This is our patient.' Because the procedure was at a technically demanding juncture, the charge nurse did not pursue the conversation further, assuming that Joan Morris had been added after the advance schedule had been distributed. Like the neurosurgery resident 90 minutes earlier, an interventional radiology doctor went to Ms Morris's room and was surprised to find it empty. He called the electrophysiology laboratory to ask why Ms Morris was undergoing this procedure. The electrophysiology doctor stated to the nurse that the call concerned a patient named Morris, but that Jane Morrison was on the table. The electrophysiology charge nurse corrected him, stating that, in fact, Joan Morris was on the table. The electrophysiology doctor asked to see the patient's chart and recognized the error.

The loss of situation awareness in this case was principally due to a series of communication failures—and at the heart of these communication failures was the absence of active identification of the patient at multiple points during her admission.

> Active patient identification (asking the patient to confirm their name, date of birth, and address, and cross-checking this against the notes or X-rays) ensures you are talking to or operating on the correct patient.

How often does wrong *site* surgery occur?

Wrong site/patient/procedure surgery can involve the:

- wrong side (left versus right)
- wrong part (wrong digit, wrong spinal level, or the wrong location within a structure—medial versus lateral, anterior versus posterior, proximal versus distal)
- wrong procedure
- wrong patient.

It is possible to operate on the correct patient, on the correct limb, and on the correct side and yet still do the wrong operation. For example, an orthopaedic surgeon might operate on the correct patient, on the correct limb (e.g. the lower limb) and on the correct side (e.g. the left side), but do the wrong procedure (a hip rather than a knee replacement—this has happened). On an operating list of three patients where there might be two hip replacements and one knee replacement scheduled, it is conceivable that he might lose situation awareness and do a knee replacement on one of the patents scheduled for a hip replacement. Such an error could occur.

What evidence we have suggests that wrong site surgery is rare occurring in between 1 in 15 500 to 1 cases of wrong site surgery per 112 994 operations.

- The JCAHO (Joint Commission on Accreditation of Healthcare Organizations) received reports on 532 sentinel events involving the wrong side, patient, or procedure surgery between 1995 and 2006. The *reported* incidence is rising.[17]

- The Physician Insurers Association of America (PIAA) has 1000 documented closed malpractice claims relating to wrong site surgery across 18 specialties in a database of 155 000 claims from 1985 to 1995.[18]

- Kwaan[19] studied malpractice claims filed between 1985 and 2003 by the Controlled Risk Insurance Corporation, a liability insurer to one-third of Massachusetts' physicians in approximately 30 hospitals). Most, though not all, cases of wrong site surgery lead to a claim, so the data represent an underestimate of the incidence of wrong site surgery. The incidence for non-spine surgery was 1 case per 112 994 operations (25 non-spine operations among a total of 2 826 367 operations, of which 12 were wrong side cases, 12 wrong site not involving laterality and one wrong patient).

- Virginia, USA—wrong site surgery was reported once in every 30 000 procedures (averaging about 1 per month).[20]

- New York State wrong site surgery is reported in every 1 in 15 500 procedures.[20]

- Orthopaedic surgeons have a 1 in 4 chance of performing a wrong site operation during a 35-year career.[21]

- Twenty-one per cent of hand surgeons report having performed at least one wrong site operation during their career, 63% of such cases involving wrong finger surgery.[22]

- Wrong site hand surgery occurs in 1 in 27 686 procedures.[22]

- In Pennsylvania, Clarke[23] identified 431 wrong site surgery cases over a 30-month period among 433 528 reports filed with the Pennsylvania Patient Safety Reporting System (PA-PSRS).
  - wrong side surgery accounted for 298 reports (70%)
  - wrong part surgery (wrong digit, wrong spinal level, etc.) accounted for 60 reports (14%)
  - wrong procedure surgery accounted for 39 reports (9%)
  - wrong patient surgery accounted for 34 reports (8%)
  - four reports involved both wrong side and wrong part (e.g. right knee versus left hip); one patient received a wrong procedure as a result of being misidentified as another patient and was counted in both categories.

How often does wrong *patient* surgery occur?

The reported frequency of wrong patient surgery depends on the methods used to collect data. Voluntary reporting systems report lower rates than mandatory ones.

Reports of sentinel events (of which wrong patient surgery is one) to the JCAHO (a voluntary reporting system) identified 17 cases over a 7-year period—roughly two cases per year.[24] The New York State mandatory reporting system received 27 reports of wrong patient procedures over a 4-year period between 1998 and 2001—roughly seven cases per year. Clarke[23] identified 34 cases of wrong patient surgery (representing 8% of all wrong site surgery in their report) over a 30-month period in Pennsylvania—roughly 12 per year.

Clarke[23] identified 39 of wrong patient surgery among 431 cases of wrong site surgery (representing 9% of all wrong site surgery) over a 30-month period.

Another real example of wrong patient surgery

The author remembers a case of a young boy who had been scheduled for removal of a cyst from inside his lower lip. The operating list was a busy one, and several other young boys were on the list, but were scheduled for circumcisions. The boy with the cyst mistakenly underwent a circumcision the mistake only being identified when his father wanted to know why the cyst on his lip was still present. The formal checking procedures in operation at the hospital in question had clearly failed to prevent the patient undergoing the wrong operation.

Wrong procedures in the non-surgical specialties

> Physicians and other non-surgeons are not immune from wrong patient procedures.

The performance of wrong patient procedures is not confined to the surgical specialties. To name but a few situations, wrong patient procedures have been reported in:

◆ communicating bad news
◆ transfusion of blood products[25]
◆ injection of radionuclide material[26]
◆ administration of chemotherapy[27]
◆ invasive cardiac electrophysiology study (the case of Joan Morrison).

> Although wrong site surgery is relatively rare, its consequences can be profound. It can occur as a consequence of operating on the wrong side, the wrong part, the wrong patient, or from doing the procedure.
>
> Surgeons are more prone to wrong patient procedures—but physicians are not immune from this error.

What surgical specialties does wrong site/wrong side surgery affect?

> No surgical specialty is immune from wrong site or wrong patient surgery.

The reported frequency of wrong site/wrong side surgery is specialty dependent. Not surprisingly, colorectal surgeons only rarely make side errors because the bulk of their work does not involve operating on a lateralized organ. However, no surgeon is immune to operating on the wrong patient or wrong doing the wrong procedure.

Some surgical specialties are at particular risk of wrong side surgery. Orthopaedic surgeons frequently operate on one or other limb and the scope for wrong side errors is greater. For hand surgeons, where there are 10 digits, there is clearly greater potential for wrong site errors. A survey of hand surgeons revealed that 21% of the respondents had operated on the wrong site at least once in their career and an additional 16% had had a near miss.[22]

- Neurosurgeons have been known to operate on the wrong side of the brain[28] and operating on the wrong spinal level is not unheard of.
- Urologists have removed the wrong kidney.
- Cardiothoracic surgeons have operated on the wrong lung.
- Gynaecologists have operated on the wrong vulva and ovary.
- Vascular surgeons have removed the wrong leg.[29]

What organs are involved with wrong site and side surgery?

Clarke reported that the following organs were involved in wrong site and wrong side surgery:

- legs, 30%
- arms, 14%

Table 7.4 In 2001 the JCAHO reported the percentage of wrong site surgery according to surgeon specialty

	%
Orthopaedic surgery	41
General surgery	20
Neurosurgery	14
Urology	11
Other surgical specialties	14

Data from root cause analysis from 126 cases of wrong site surgery in a JCAHO database.[30]

- head and neck structures, 24%
- genitourinary, pelvic, or groin structures, 21%
- lumbar structures, 7%
- chest, 6%
- breast, 3%.

In this particular study no wrong site errors involved the heart, liver, biliary system, pancreas, or spleen.

Why does wrong site/wrong side surgery occur?

The JCAHO has identified **communication errors** and **failure to comply with procedures** (e.g. not following the 'rules' of cross-referencing to other information sources) as the two most common causes of wrong site surgery.

There is no one single cause for wrong site or wrong patient surgery. The main causes are communication errors and not following procedures that reduce such errors:

- communication errors and poor communication between members of the operating team
- failure to engage the patient (or family where appropriate) in the process of identifying the correct site/side
- no or inadequate verification checklist in the anaesthetic room and/or operating theatre (to ensure all relevant information sources are cross-checked against the patient's identity)
- failure to review the medical records or imaging studies in the immediate pre-operative period
- relying solely on a single healthcare worker to check the side and site, e.g. sole reliance on the surgeon to check
- absence of any verbal communication in the checking procedure
- operation site and side unclear from notes.

A substantial proportion of surgeons do not follow recommended methods for the prevention of wrong site/side surgery, e.g. only 30% of orthopaedic surgeons followed recommendations for eliminating wrong site/side surgery in a survey conducted in 2000.[31]

Surgeons and other operating team have a variety of excuses for not performing safety checks to prevent wrong site and wrong patient surgery, all of which we have heard:

- 'We check anyway'
- 'Its another piece of paper to fill in'

- 'There's already too much paperwork'
- 'We'd never make such a basic error'
- 'Let the resident do it'
- 'Put the patient to sleep—I'll be right there'.

We are not perfect—in the past one of us has been heard to use the latter phrase!

Barriers to prevention of wrong site/wrong side surgery

- *Multiple* different checking systems are a barrier to safety (as opposed to a *limited* number of checking systems).
- Standard operating procedures (*standardized* across an organization) enhance safety.

High reliability organizations adopt so-called standard operating procedures—a single method of performing a particular task. In the NHS there is no one standard method for preventing wrong site or wrong patient surgery. The Royal College of Surgeons (RCS) and the National Patient Safety Agency have proposed one such standardized scheme, but it is not mandatory for NHS organizations to use it and it has imperfections that make it difficult to use. One of the authors operates in two different NHS Hospital Trusts—in one he is required to use the form, but in the other he is not! The RCS/NPSA checking process consists of a four-point checklist that requires four signatures on a form, the so-called 'preoperative marking checklist' (Fig. 7.3). The checking process starts on the ward and proceeds through to the point immediately prior to commencement of the operation.

This rather protracted checking process is perceived by some staff as cumbersome and onerous ('yet another piece of paper to complete', 'loads of signatures required'). Making something difficult to complete *increases* the likelihood that it will not be completed in the way that was intended. The theatre nursing staff are required to ensure that the form is completed—they run the risk of being disciplined if it is not. One of the authors has seen nurses asking surgeons to complete the form *after* the operation has been completed solely to avoid disciplinary action. The purpose of signing the form, therefore, becomes the avoidance of disciplinary action rather than its supposed primary purpose as a safety measure to avoid wrong site surgery. Some surgeons sign all of their sections of the form *before* the patient even gets into the anaesthetic room (again defeating the purpose of the checklist), to 'save time'. Thus, the form's purpose as far as some theatre nurses and doctors are concerned is to

Check 1 (the operating surgeon, or nominated deputy, who will be present in the theatre at the time of the patient's procedure)

♦ Check the patient's identity and wrist band

♦ Check reliable documentation and images to ascertain intended surgical site

♦ Mark the intended site with an arrow using an indelible pen

Check 2 (ward or day care staff)

♦ Before leaving the ward check the patient's identity and wristband, inspect the mark and confirm against the patient's supporting documentation

♦ Relevant imaging studies must accompany the patient or be available in the operating theatre suite

Check 3 (operating surgeon or a senior member of the surgical team)

♦ In the anaesthetic room and prior to anaesthesia, check the patient's identity and wristband, inspect the mark and check against the patient's supporting documentation

♦ Re-check imaging studies accompany patient or are available in operating theatre

♦ The availability of the correct implant (if applicable)

Check 4 (theatre staff directly involved in the intended operative procedure; the 'scrub nurse')

♦ The surgical, anaesthetic and theatre team involved in the intended operative procedure prior to commencement of surgery should pause for verbal briefing to confirm:

♦ Presence of the correct patient

♦ Marking of the correct site

♦ Procedure to be performed

Fig. 7.3 The RCS/NPSA checking process consists of a four-point checklist that requires four signatures on a form, the so-called 'Preoperative marking checklist' (the staff with responsibility for each action are shown in brackets).

act as a piece of paper on which a series of signatures must be obtained rather than a mechanism to prevent wrong patient and wrong site surgery.

The requirement for the surgical, anaesthetic, and theatre team involved in the operation to pause for a verbal briefing to confirm the correct patient, the correct site, and the correct procedure is often not (maybe never) done. So the form remains a form on which a series of signatures must be obtained and nothing more!

So, site-verification protocols may not be being followed at least partly because of the complexity of some current systems—operating teams are human and the more complex a site-verification protocol the less user friendly will it be. When it comes to pre-operative checklists, the KISS principle (Keep it Simple) is better than the KICK principle (Keep it Complicated).

Barriers to prevention of wrong site/wrong side surgery include:

◆ many different types of verification protocols
◆ protocols that do not involve the patient
◆ multiple (as opposed to a limited number of) personnel required to complete the checking protocol
◆ multiple *separate* checking steps by *disparate* individuals or groups of individuals—the nurses do their check, the anaesthetist does his or her check, the surgeon does his or her check, but none of the three teams do a *combined* check
◆ complex checklists that requirement multiple signatures
◆ checking procedure that is non-verbal.

Can wrong site/wrong side/wrong patient surgery be prevented?

On the face of it this seems a strange question to ask. Surely the answer must be yes—of course we can prevent it and we should be able to prevent *all* such cases. Surely to suggest otherwise is defeatist. However, no system is ideal.

◆ Kwaan[19] estimates that only 62% of wrong site surgery could have been prevented using the JCAHO Universal Protocol for site verification; 38% would not have been prevented.
◆ Clarke[23] found that a formal time-out procedure was unsuccessful in preventing wrong surgery in 31 cases (7%) among 427 wrong site operations—a so-called 'time-out failure'.

Thus reliance on a single safety system—carefully designed though that system may be—is flawed. An example of such a system can be found in the bolt that attaches the rotor of a Huey helicopter to the body of the helicopter (Fig. 7.4). If this bolt fails, the helicopter will crash, hence the nickname of 'Jesus bolt' given to the bolt by US aircrew who flew these helicopters during the Vietnam war. The safety of the entire helicopter is critically dependent on this bolt. 'Jesus bolts' are frequently found in healthcare situations.

However, having too many checking procedures is also counter-productive.

There is a happy balance of more than one checking procedure (avoiding the Jesus bolt analogy), but not too many (because humans get bored when they have to go through a whole raft of checking procedures).

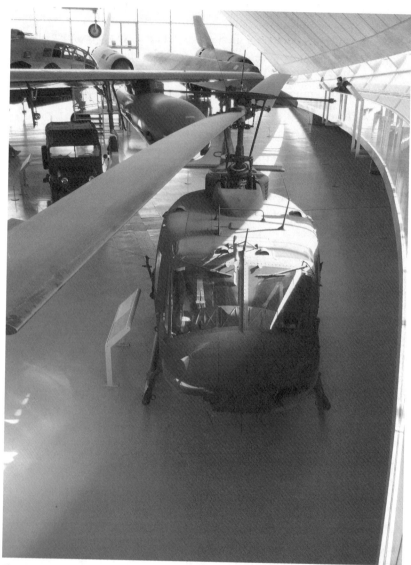

Fig. 7.4 The rotor of this Huey helicopter is held in place by a single bolt. If this bolt fails, the helicopter will crash, hence the nickname of 'Jesus bolt' given to the bolt by US aircrew who flew these helicopters during the Vietnam war (®Oxford Urology Courses, Permission granted).

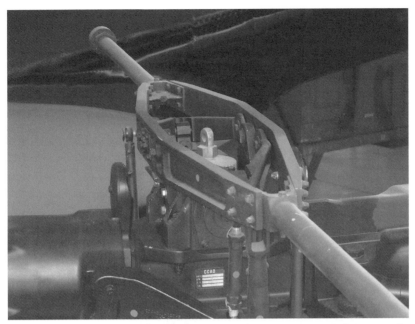

Fig. 7.5 A close up of the 'Jesus bolt' (®Oxford Urology Courses, Permission granted).

The UK-based medical insurance company, The Medical Defence Union (MDU) has issued specific advice on how to reduce the risk of wrong site/wrong patient surgery.[32]

- **Avoid abbreviations** when referring to site, side, or anatomical location, in written notes, consent forms, and on operating lists. Digits of the hand should be described as the thumb, index, middle, ring or little finger; those of the foot as the hallux, second, third, fourth, fifth toes.
- **Use multiple sources of written information** to confirm that you are doing the correct operation on the correct side and in the correct patient (e.g. the original referral letter, the notes, consent form, and X-rays).
- **Mark** the site and side of the operation (a member of the surgical team who is going to be present at the operation).
- The process of marking should involve **more than one** member of clinical staff and preferably the patient or a family member.
- **Involve the patient** when marking: (a) actively identify them ('just confirm your address and date of birth'), and (b) 'tell me what operation you're having today and what side we're operating on'.

- Use a clear, unambiguous, **indelible pen** to mark the site.
- As the operating surgeon you should **see the patient before administration of anaesthesia**. Ensure that all clinical documentation is available (referral letter, source of referral, a signed consent form, supporting radiological images).
- Double check the site when the patient is on the operating table, and **before** draping.
- Make sure the mark is **clearly visible** after the drapes have been positioned.
- Take a '**time-out**' before the procedure starts to confirm the patient details and the site and side of the operation against the clinical records.

How can wrong site/wrong side surgery be prevented?

There is no one single cause and, therefore, there is no one single solution.

Prevention of wrong site surgery—first and foremost do not rely on any single method—use a limited* number of checks.
(*Many different checking procedures are, paradoxically, a barrier to safety as they confuse staff and reduce compliance. Two checking systems, for example, is safer than one, but is also safer than half a dozen different checking systems.)

Site and patient verification protocols are the foundation for preventing wrong site and wrong patient surgery, but other checks are required if all such cases are to be prevented.

In the same way that we nowadays regard taking consent as a process, rather than an event, try to think about the procedure for ensuring the correct patient, correct site and side, and correct procedure as a *process*, not as a single *event*.

The process should involve the following:

- a pre-procedure review by the doctor who will do the procedure (not a deputy)—this is the *initial* step in the process of confirmation of correct patient, procedure, etc.
- mark the site and side with an indelible marker—avoid placing the mark such that an imprint of the wet ink could be transferred to the opposite side or a different site.
- A verification step in the anaesthetic room by the surgeon and another responsible healthcare worker such as the anaesthetist, involving a review of relevant documentation (notes, consent form, radiology test results*).

◆ A final time-out immediately before the operation, when the patient has been positioned on the operating table, using a formal checklist with another healthcare worker (e.g. anaesthetist) to confirm patient identity, planned procedure, and site and side of that procedure*).

(*Involvement of others—nurses, anaesthetist, operating department assistants, anaesthetic nurses—is a crucial step to site and side safety. Each member of the team brings their own situation awareness (their own perception of the plan) to the team—as a result team situation awareness is created. The chances of an individual committing an error in the site/side/patient/procedure checking process is greater than several members of the team committing the same error—as long as the team members check *together*.)

> ### Teams make smarter decisions than individuals
>
> Do not rely on a single piece of documentation or a single person to do the check—involve other members of the team as it is unlikely that the same error will be repeated by every team member involved in the checking process.

First, do not rely on a single piece of information to confirm the operative site and side—refer to the notes, the X-rays, letters of correspondence and, of course, confirm the site/side with the patient. The patient won't always know (e.g. a kidney cancer may have caused no symptoms at all and may only have been identified radiologically as an incidental finding), but in many cases the patient will have had symptoms referable to a specific site or side:

Which hip has been the one that's bothering you?

Which finger is the troublesome one?

Which side has the pain been on?

Marking the operative site

◆ The mark should be made by the operating surgeon, rather than by someone who is not going to be present during the operation
◆ Use an indelible marker—avoid placing the mark such that an imprint of the wet ink could be transferred to the opposite side or a different site
◆ Sign your site—put your initials on the appropriate site
◆ Avoid abbreviations—write 'LEFT' or 'RIGHT'
◆ The mark must be visible after the patient has been prepped and draped

Take a 'time-out' immediately before the procedure

A final verification (with reference to the notes and X-rays) with other staff members, e.g. the anaesthetist and scrub nurse.

In the USA this process has been summarized by The Joint Commission on Accreditation of Healthcare Organization in its 'Universal Protocol to prevent wrong site surgery' (Fig. 7.6).

Remember

- No one single method will prevent all wrong site/side/patient or procedure errors
- Errors can still be made after the side has been marked
- Errors can still be made despite the use of a time-out procedure
- A time-out in the anaesthetic room combined with a time-out once the patient is positioned on the operating table may reduce wrong site, side, patient, and procedure errors

---

Wrong site surgery can be prevented by a process of two (or more) health-care workers simultaneously performing a verbal process (preferably using a checklist) of cross-checking the patient's identity against at least one other source of information (such as the patient's notes, X-rays, consent form—or indeed by asking the patient themselves prior to induction of anaesthesia).

Wrong site, wrong patient, wrong procedure surgery prevention: summary[33]

- A process—not an event
- Involve the patient in the process
- Create an atmosphere and develop procedures where all the team members can share their 'individual situation awareness'
- Cross-check with the consent form and notes
- Have a formal time-out prior to each procedure as a final check.

Involve your patients in ensuring correct site and side surgery In the USA, patients are encouraged to be involved in the process of ensuring that they get the correct operation, on the correct side. While some of the advice given in 'Tips for patients to prevent wrong site surgery' is clearly relevant only to a US 'audience', much of the advice could easily be adapted to your practice and your patients.

Wrong site, wrong procedure, wrong person surgery can be prevented. This universal protocol is intended to achieve that goal. It is based on the consensus of experts from the relevant clinical specialties and professional disciplines and is endorsed by more than 40 professional medical associations and organizations. In developing this protocol, consensus was reached on the following principles:

◆ wrong site, wrong procedure, wrong person surgery can and must be prevented.

◆ a robust approach—using multiple, complementary strategies—is necessary to achieve the goal of eliminating wrong site, wrong procedure, wrong person surgery.

◆ active involvement and effective communication among all members of the surgical team is important for success.

◆ to the extent possible, the patient (or legally designated representative) should be involved in the process.

◆ consistent implementation of a standardized approach using a universal, consensus-based protocol will be most effective.

◆ the protocol should be flexible enough to allow for implementation with appropriate adaptation when required to meet specific patient needs.

◆ a requirement for site marking should focus on cases involving right/left distinction, multiple structures (fingers, toes), or levels (spine).

◆ the universal protocol should be applicable or adaptable to all operative and other invasive procedures that expose patients to harm, including procedures done in settings other than the operating room.

In concert with these principles, the following steps, taken together, comprise the Universal Protocol for eliminating wrong site, wrong procedure, wrong person surgery:

◆ *Pre-operative verification process*

Purpose: to ensure that all of the relevant documents and studies are available before the start of the procedure and that they have been reviewed and are consistent with each other and with the patient's expectations and with the team's understanding of the intended patient, procedure, site, and, as applicable, any implants. Missing information or discrepancies must be addressed before starting the procedure.

Process: an ongoing process of information gathering and verification, beginning with the determination to do the procedure, continuing through all settings and interventions involved in the pre-operative preparation of the patient, up to and including the 'time-out' just before the start of the procedure.

◆ *Marking the operative site*

Purpose: to identify unambiguously the intended site of incision or insertion.

Process: for procedures involving right/left distinction, multiple structures (such as fingers and toes), or multiple levels (as in spinal procedures), the intended site must be marked such that the mark will be visible after the patient has been prepped and draped.

◆ *'Time-out' immediately before starting the procedure*

Purpose: to conduct a final verification of the correct patient, procedure, site and, as applicable, implants.

Process: active communication among all members of the surgical/procedure team, consistently initiated by a designated member of the team, conducted in a 'fail-safe' mode, i.e., the procedure is not started until any questions or concerns are resolved.

©The Joint Commission, 2008 (Reprinted with permission)
http://www.jointcommission.org/NR/rdonlyres/E3C600EB-043B-4E86-B04E-
CA4A89AD5433/0/universal_protocol.pdf.

Fig. 7.6 The Universal Protocol to prevent wrong site surgery of the Joint Commission on Accreditation of Healthcare Organization.

- You and your surgeon should agree on exactly what will be done during the operation.

- Ask to have the surgical site marked with a permanent marker and to be involved in marking the site. This means that the site cannot be easily overlooked or confused (for example, surgery on the right knee instead of the left knee).

- Ask questions. You should speak up if you have concerns. It's okay to ask questions and expect answers that you understand.

- Think of yourself as an active participant in the safety and quality of your healthcare. Studies show that patients who are actively involved in making decisions about their care are more likely to have good outcomes.

- Insist that your surgery be done at a Joint Commission-accredited facility. Joint Commission accreditation is considered the 'gold standard,' meaning that the hospital or surgery center has undergone a rigorous on-site evaluation and is committed to national quality and safety standards.

(With permission from The Joint Commission on
Accreditation of Healthcare Organization).
© The Joint Commission, 2008. Reprinted with permission.
http://www.jointcommission.org/PatientSafety/
UniversalProtocol/wss_tips.htm/.)

Fig. 7.7 Tips for patients to prevent wrong site surgery.

Much of this can be incorporated into a checklist. Checklists formalize the process of carrying out the pre-procedure checks, and, thereby, are a way of ensuring that parts of the process are not omitted (**BEWARE**—they do not guarantee prevention of omission of vital steps).

Two examples of so-called 'Call and Response' Checklists are shown in Figs 7.8 and 7.9 (**The Exeter checklist**). **The Oxford Checklist** is printed on a laminated A4 sheet and the Exeter Checklist on a large (A3 size) sheet of laminated paper posted on to the wall of the operating theatre. The checklists are 'called' and 'responded' to verbally by the surgeon and the anaesthetist. This process means that no additional paperwork is generated. The procedure for completion of each checklist is as follows.

When the patient is stable on the table and immediately before the surgical scrub, the surgeon calls for the checklist to be read. The surgeon holds the patient's notes in one hand and he positions the patient's wrist in such a way as to be able to read the identity bracelet. The anaesthetist holds the consent form and drug chart.

The anaesthetist 'calls'	The surgeon 'responds'
Anaesthetist holds consent form and drug chart	*Surgeon holds notes and patient's identity bracelet*
Patient's name and date of birth	Name _____
	Date of birth _____
What operation are you doing?	I'm doing a (*name of operation*)
If lateralized procedure anaesthetist and surgeon cross to computer screen to view images	*Surgeon checks side with X-rays and report* .
What side are you operating on?	I'm operating on the (*announce side*) side
Return to patient—surgeon calls	**Return to patient—anaesthetist checks anaesthetic chart and 'responds'**
What antibiotic and what dose have you given?	I have given (*state type and dose*)
Are the TED stockings on?	The TED stockings are on
What dose of heparin have you given?	I have given 5000 units of subcut heparin
Are the flotrons in place and switched on?	The flotrons are in place and are switched on

Fig. 7.8 A 'call and response' pre-procedure checklist used in The Department of Urology in Oxford. The anaesthetist and urologist complete this checklist when the patient has been stabilised on the operating table, prior to commencement of the surgical scrub.

Time out

Key: anaesthestist text   surgeon text

Anaesthetist hold consent form and drug chart	Surgeon holds notes and id bracelet
Patient's name and DOB	Name ....
	Date of birth ....
What operation are you doing?	I'm doing a ....
Are there potential problems?	Potential problems are ....
Which side are you operating on?	I'm operating on the .... side
Surgeon demonstrates side on PACS screen to anaesthetist	
What antibiotic have you given?	I have given..
Has Heparin been given?	Heparin was given ....
Are TED stockings on?	TED stockings are on ....

Fig. 7.9 The Exeter checklist (a modification of the Oxford checklist). Another example of a 'call and response' pre-procedure checklist. Reproduced courtesy of Mr Richard Berrisford, Royal Devon and Exeter Foundation NHS Trust.

The anaesthetist calls for the name and date of birth of the patient. The surgeon reads out loud the name and date of birth of the patient from the notes and checks that this is the same as on the identity bracelet. The anaesthetist checks that the same name and date of birth is on the consent form and drug chart.

The anaesthetist then calls for the name of the procedure and the surgeon announces this while checking that this is consistent with the notes. He may physically point to the words on the page. The anaesthetist checks that the stated procedure is given on the consent form.

In the Exeter Checklist the anaesthetist then asks if there are any potential problems. This is an opportunity for the surgeon to remind himself of the case and to give a short briefing to the surgical team about any special conditions related to this particular operation. These might include:

- contingencies
- abnormalities
- previous medical history
- drugs given to the patient
- availability of implants
- availability and serviceability of instruments and special equipment
- the presence of and duties of any new members of the surgical team.

If this is a procedure where there is a possibility of making a wrong side or site error, the anaesthetist asks 'which side will you be operating on?' The surgeon uses the X-rays and radiologist's report to confirm the side, pointing to the laterality markers on the X-ray film and the appropriate words in the radiologist's report (e.g. 'right side renal tumour').

At this point the anaesthetist and surgeon swap the 'calling' and 'response' roles. The surgeon now makes the calls with the anaesthetist responding. The surgeon asks the anaesthetist if the antibiotics and heparin have been given and if the TED stockings are on.

In straightforward cases, without abnormal surgical conditions requiring a special briefing, the checklist can be usually carried out in less than 60 seconds. No additional paperwork is required. The whole process is verbalized.

An additional 'layer' of safety can be included by the announcement by the surgeon of 'Pre-operative checklist complete'. There have been instances in aviation where there was an interruption during the checklist reading and the team were distracted and forgot that the checklist had not been completed. They then carried on with the activity with a crucial element not in place.

Announcing checklist complete provides **'memorability'** and may help to prevent the team being uncertain whether or not they have done things.

The requirement for an audit trail can be satisfied by one member of the surgical team who has no immediate task at that instant (possibly a theatre nurse) writing a note in the patient's records: 'Pre-operative checklist completed'.

Situation awareness and retained swabs and surgical instruments

Incidence

This is difficult to determine. It may occur at least once per year in a hospital performing between 8000 and 18 000 major operations per year.[34] Incidence rates tend to be based on claims data and, therefore, are likely to underestimate the true scale of the problem because not all cases end in litigation (though many do). The rates of retained swabs are higher in:

- emergency surgery
- unexpected change in surgical procedure
- higher body mass index.

Anatomical sites of retained swabs and instruments[35]

- Abdominal cavity
- Chest
- Pelvis
- Vagina.

Consequences

Asymptomatic Retained swabs and instruments may be asymptomatic. There was a surge in incidence of retained swabs and instruments around 2001 after the commencement of heightened security at airports following the 9/11 terrorist attacks. Patients with retained instruments triggered metal detectors at airport security check points.

Symptomatic Acute injury leading to early presentation, e.g. bowel perforation, bladder perforation, vessels perforation—haemorrhage.

Delayed reaction

- Fistula formation between an organ and skin (e.g. an enterocutaneous fistula).
- Encapsulation of the retained swab or instrument in fibrous tissue leading to development of a mass that can cause, for example, a bowel obstruction.

Prevention protocols[36]

- Use a standardized counting procedure.
- Explore the wound or body cavity before closure.
- Avoid relying on just one aspect of sensory perception—**SEE** *AND* **TOUCH**.
- Abdomen and pelvis—systematically examine all four quadrants; look between loops of bowel; examine anatomical recesses; look where retractor blades were placed; look behind the bladder and uterus.
- Examine the vagina if entered or explored.
- In the chest—examine the retrocardiac space; elevate the apex of the heart and look in the transverse sinus to the right and left of the aorta and pulmonary artery; examine the apices and bases of the thoracic cavity.
- Use only X-ray detectable items in the surgical wound/body cavity.
- Consider the use of plastic hanging counting device.

What to do if there is an incorrect count

- **STOP CLOSING THE WOUND**—be patient with your scrub nurse—she is trying to help your patient and you.
- If necessary remove wound closure sutures to allow better access to the wound for inspection and palpation.
- Replace retractors if necessary to assist exposure.
- Repeat your systematic examination of all sites within the wound or body cavity.

References

1 **Endsley M.** Situation awareness global assessment technique. Proceedings of the Aerospace and Electronics Conference, 1988.
2 **Endsley M.** Toward a theory of situation awareness in dynamic systems. *Hum Factors* 1995; **37**: 32–64.
3 **Tan K-W, Kaber DB, Riley J, Endsley MR.** Human factors issues in the implementation of adaptive automation in complex systems In: *The proceedings of the XIVth triennial congress of the International Ergonomics Association and 44th annual meeting of the Human Factors and Ergonomics Society.* Santa Monica, CA: Human Factors and Ergonomics Society; 2000: pp. 97–100.
4 **Adam EC.** Fighter cockpits of the future. *Proceedings of 12th IEEE/AIAA Digital Avionics Systems Conference (DASC)* 1993; 318–23.
5 **Jeannot E, Kelly C, Thompson D.** *the development of situation awareness measures in air traffic management systems.* Brussels: Eurocontrol; 2003.
6 **Moray N.** Ou sont les neiges d'antan? ('Where are the snows of yesteryear?'). In: *Human performance, situation awareness and automation: current research and trends* (eds DA Vincenzi, M Mouloua, PA Hancock). Lawrence Erlbaum, Philadelphia, USA, 2004; pp. 1–31.

7 Rabardel P. (1995). *Les Hommes et les Technologies: approche cognitive des instruments contemporains*. Paris: A. Colin 1995.

8 Vincent C (ed.). *Clinical risk management: enhancing patient safety*, 2nd edn. London: BMJ Books; 2001.

9 Besnard D, Greathead D. When mental models go wrong. Co-occurences in dynamic, critical systems. *Int J Hum Comput Stud* 2004; **60**: 117–28.

10 Luchins A. Primacy-recency in impression formation. In *The order of presentation in persuasion* (ed. CI Holland). New Haven, CT: Yale University Press; 1957: pp. 33–61.

11 Rasmussen J, Vicente KJ. Coping with human errors through system design: implications for ecological interface design. *Int J Man-Machine Stud* 1989; **31**: 517–34.

12 Mazur A. Three Mile Island and the scientific community. *Ann N Y Acad Sci* 1981; **365**: 216–21.

13 Anderson CA, Lepper MR, Ross L. Perseverance of social theories: the role of explanation in the persistence of discredited information. *J Pers Soc Psychol* 1980; **39**: 1037–49.

14 Hawkins F. *Human factors in flight*. Aldershot: Ashgate Publishing.

15 The human factor: the critical importance of effective teamwork and communication in providing safe care: M Leonard, S Graham and D Bonacum—Qual Saf Healthcare 2004 13- i85—i90

16 'Derail' Darlow Smithson TV Programme. http://www.darlowsmithson.com/.

17 http://www.jointcommission.org/NR/rdonlyres/67297896–4E16–4BB7-BF0F-5DA4A87B02F2/0/se_stats_trends_year.pdf

18 Shojania KG, Duncan BW, McDonald KM, *et al*. Agency for Healthcare Research and Quality. *Making healthcare safer: a critical analysis of patient safety practices. Strategies to avoid wrong-site surgery*. Evidence Report/Technology Assessment No.43, AHRQ Publication No. 01-E058. Rockville MD: Agency for Healthcare Research and Quality; 2001: pp. 498–503.

19 Kwaan MR, Studdert DM, Zinner MJ, *et al*. Incidence, patterns, and prevention of wrong-site surgery. *Arch Surg* 2006; **141**: 353–7.

20 Dunn D. Surgical site verification: A through Z. *J Perianesth* 2006; **21**: 317–31.

21 Canale ST. Wrong-site surgery: a preventable complication. *Clin Orthop Relat Res* 2005; **433**: 26–9.

22 Meinberg EG, Stern PJ. Incidence of wrong-site surgery among hand surgeons. *J Bone Joint Surg* 2003; **85A**: 193–7.

23 Clarke JR, Johnston J, Finley ED. Getting surgery right. *Ann Surg* 2007; **246**: 395–403.

24 Chassin MR, Becher EC. The wrong patient. *Ann Intern Med* 2002; **136**: 826–33.

25 Linden JV, Paul B, Dressler KP. A report of 104 transfusion errors in New York State. *Transfusion* 1992; **32**: 601–6.

26 Serig DI. Radiopharmaceutical misadministrations: What's wrong? In: *Human error in medicine* (ed. MS Bogner). Hillsdale, NJ: Lawrence Erlbaum Associates; 1994: pp. 179–96.

27 Schulmeister L. Chemotherapy medication errors: descriptions, severity and contributing factors. *Oncol Nurs Forum* 1999; **26**: 1033–42.

28 Meakins JL. Site and side of surgery: getting it right. *Can J Surg* 2003; **46**: 85–7.

29 Crane M. When a surgical mistake becomes a media event. *Med Econ* 1997; **16**: 44–51.

30 Joint Commission on Accreditation of Health Care Organizations 2001. http://www.jointcommission.org/

31 OK plan to end wrong-site surgeries. American Academy of Orthopaedic Surgeons (AAOS). *AAOS Bull* http://www.aaos.org/wordhtml/ bulletin/oct97/wrong.htm/.

32 http://www.the-mdu.com/

33 American College of Surgeons [ST-41]. *Statement on ensuring correct patient, correct site and correct procedure surgery.* http://www.facs.org/fellows_info/statements/st-41.html. Accessed on 1.1.09.

34 Gawande AA, Studdert DM, Orav EJ, *et al.* Risk factors for retained instruments and sponges after surgery. *N Engl J Med* 2003; **348**: 229–35.

35 Kaiser CW, Friedman S, Spurling KP, *et al.* The retained surgical sponge. *Ann Surg* 1996; **224**: 79–84.

36 http://www.facs.org/fellows-info/bulletin/2005/gibbs/1005.pdf

Further reading

Association of PeriOperative Registered Nurses. *Recommended practices for sponge, sharp and instrument counts in AORN standards, recommended practices and guidelines.* Denver, CO: AORN, Inc.; 2004.

Bernstein M. Wrong-side surgery: systems for prevention. *Can J Surg* 2003; **46**: 144–6.

Correct patient, correct site and correct procedure surgery. *Bull Am Coll Surg* 2002; **87**: 26.

Fabian C. Electronic tagging of surgical sponges to prevent their accidental retention. *Surgery* 2005; **137**: 298–301.

Gibbs VC, Auerbach AD. The retained surgical sponge. In: *Making healthcare safer: a critical analysis of patient safety practices* (eds Shojania KG, Duncan BW, McDonald KM, Wachter RM). Rockville, MD: Agency for Healthcare Research and Quality; 2001: pp. 255–7.

Lewis BD. *Guidelines to reduce the incidence of wrong level spinal surgery.* http://www.coa-aco.org/library/health_policy/guidelines_to_reduce_the_indidence_of_wrong_level_spinal_surgery.html

O'Connor AR, Coakley FV, Meng MV, *et al.* Imaging of retained surgical sponges in the abdomen and pelvis. *Am J Roentgenol* 2003; **180**: 481–9.

Sandlin D. Surgichip—new technology for prevention of wrong site, wrong procedure, wrong person surgery. *J Perianesth Nurs* 2005; **20**: 144–6.

Useful websites

www.ihi.org—Institute for Healthcare Improvement.

www.ama-assn.org/—National Patient Safety Foundation (at the AMA).

www.ahcpr.gov—Agency for Healthcare Policy and Research (AHCPR).

www.aorn.org—Association of Operating Room Nurses (AORN).

www.jacho.org—Joint Commission on Accreditation of Healthcare Organizations.

Chapter 8

Professional culture

In 1954, the actor James Robertson Justice was cast to play the role of Sir Lancelot Spratt in the film version of Richard Gordon's *Doctor in the house*. The bearded actor had a domineering personality, an irascible character, a bulky physique, and a commanding voice. He was clearly the type of surgeon who knew no fear in the face of torrential haemorrhage. His caricature of the senior doctor was seen by many to be an accurate portrayal of many senior doctors they knew and reflected the professional culture of medicine and surgery.

A year later Justice was also cast to play the role of a senior pilot, Captain Douglas Brent in the film *Out of the clouds* set at the newly opened Heathrow airport. Many pilots recognized in Justice's performance the arrogant manner of the 'Atlantic Baron', a member of the group of senior pilots who flew the prestigious transatlantic flights to the USA.

In both films Justice employs an identical characterization. He sweeps through St Swithin's hospital or Heathrow airport booming out instructions to scurrying minions. He makes sarcastic remarks even to those who answer him correctly. In both films he forcefully reminds stunned subordinates that he is always right and that he has carried out more gastrectomies or crossed the Atlantic more times than anyone else.

The fact that Justice was able to use an identical characterization to represent both a senior doctor and a senior pilot reflected similarities in the two professional cultures.

Similarities between two professions

Both doctors and pilots operate in safety-critical domains where situations are often complex and counter-intuitive and where it takes many years of training and experience to deal with a wide range of scenarios and hazards.

The two professions adopted a 'macho' or masculine culture with powerful individuals wanting to be seen to be demonstrating courage and high levels of technical competence.

Another similarity between the two professions is that both work closely with another profession that has a predominantly 'feminine' or 'caring' culture.

Doctors work with nurses, and pilots work with cabin crew (once a predominantly female occupation). It is possible that this cultural interface reinforced the macho behaviours of both the doctors and pilots.

Negative aspects of professional cultures

A professional culture has both positive and negative aspects. A group of well-intentioned, well-trained people can still produce harm if they happen to be working in a culture that lacks candour and insight into its own shortcomings.

As the final report of Professor Kennedy's inquiry into the care of children receiving complex heart surgery at the Bristol Royal Infirmary observed:[1]

> The story of the paediatric cardiac surgical service in Bristol is not an account of bad people. Nor is it an account of people who did not care, nor of people who wilfully harmed patients.
>
> It is an account of people who cared greatly about human suffering, and were dedicated and well-motivated. Sadly, some lacked insight and their behaviour was flawed. Many failed to communicate with each other, and to work together effectively for the interests of their patients. There was a lack of leadership, and of teamwork.

The report concluded that approximately 30 children who underwent heart surgery at the Bristol Royal Infirmary between 1991 and 1995 died unnecessarily as a result of substandard care.

Steep hierarchy

Another observation made in the Kennedy report[1] was that there was:

> an imbalance of power, with too much control in the hands of a few individuals

An imbalance of power in a culture can result in a 'steep hierarchy'.

It might seem convenient to a busy senior operator to have his juniors carry out his instructions without question. However, the Elaine Bromiley case and three others in Chapter 4 (case studies 5, 7, and 20) could have been prevented if a junior had questioned his senior's actions and had spoken up. The experience of the aviation industry has been that several major disasters have occurred where juniors had not been sufficiently assertive.

> In some airline accidents the psychological pressure preventing the co-pilot from confronting the captain was so great that the co-pilot failed to speak up in the face of an evolving accident.

As a consequence the co-pilot, the captain, the cabin crew, and all the passengers died.

The psychological pressure preventing speaking up can therefore be immense.

In all of these cases with the benefit of hindsight the team leader must have bitterly regretted that the junior had not been more assertive when they realized a serious error had been made.

In addition to inhibiting the detection of incipient adverse events, a steep hierarchy can also lead to long-term system failures where potential adverse events are not addressed.

During a patient safety course at one hospital in London a video was shown about an adverse event where the mouth and lips of a 4-year-old boy were badly burned during a maxillofacial procedure, as a consequence of a *dry* swab catching fire during the application of diathermy.

One of the delegates on the patient safety course that day was the lead maxillofacial surgeon of the hospital. The potential for such a fire risk had not occurred to him before and he always used dry swabs. During the afternoon coffee break he went back to his department to make enquiries and found that the other consultant did know of the danger and always took the precaution of dampening swabs in saline solution. As a result, from 3 p.m. that afternoon the maxillofacial department of that hospital adopted the standard operating procedure of using moistened swabs.

Later the consultant asked his theatre nurses why they had never pointed out that the two consultants in the department were using different procedures. One said she did not think it was her place to give *him* any advice. Another said she had once tried to make a similar observation some years before to a consultant and had received such a response from him that she never offered any safety suggestions ever again.

Thus a steep hierarchy can make nurses and junior doctors too unassertive. A toxic culture is created that produces other harmful problems, such as bullying. An article by Lyn Quine in the *British Medical Journal*[2] on bullying in an NHS trust described the results of a staff questionnaire survey. The article concluded that bullying is a serious problem in the NHS. Over one-third of the participants in the survey (38%) reported experiencing one or more types of bullying in the previous year. Forty-two per cent had witnessed the bullying of others. The remedy for this problem lies in facilitating more assertive behaviours.

At the senior doctor level, however, the professional hierarchy can be too flat. The Medical Director of a hospital might find it difficult to obtain complete compliance if he were to order senior doctors in his hospital to adopt a new standard procedure such as the use of 'read back' or pre-operative checklists. In contrast in a similar situation in aviation if the Chief Pilot decided to introduce a new standard procedure, he would explain the reasons behind his decision and his instructions would be followed without complaint.

The pilots' professional culture also at one time had features that either directly induced adverse events or prevented measures from being taken to mitigate them. Over the last 30 years a range of measures have been taken to modify the hazardous attitudes and behaviours of airline pilots. Some of these measures could be introduced into healthcare. It might be of interest to doctors to understand how cultural changes were effected in aviation.

Changing the pilots' professional culture

In the 1970s and 1980s a series of major accidents occurred around the world to large passenger jet aircraft. These crashes cost the industry approximately $10 billion and the loss of some 7000 lives. In most cases, investigators were confident that the aircraft had been entirely serviceable prior to the impact and that no 'technical factor' had caused the accident. They were also able to exclude bad weather as a causative factor. Clearly, some type of 'pilot error' or 'human factor' had been responsible.

The airline industry began to realize that it had very little understanding of the nature of human error and that as a consequence there was no likelihood of finding an immediate solution. It did not seem to occur to aviation industry leaders to approach either academia or other professions or industries for advice as flying was believed to be such a unique venture that there would be no parallels in any other industry's experiences.

The measures that were adopted included:

- standard operating procedures—followed very closely and consistently
- creation of a 'less steep' hierarchy through crew resource management training
- use of simulators to develop teamwork skills
- acceptance of auditing.

Standard operating procedures

In order to try to understand the nature of pilot error, airliner cockpits were fitted with microphones connected to tape recorders in the 'black box' to record conversations in the cockpit. Within a few years the industry had acquired a dozen or so recordings of the crews' interactions immediately before an accident.

Having studied these, it became clear that in almost all cases, there had been a lack of co-ordination in the crews' activities. In some cases the co-pilots had seemed not to have understood what the captain was doing. Different captains often carried out the same flight manoeuvres in different ways and this variation seemed to have delayed the timely detection of errors by the co-pilots.

Some airlines responded to these problems by adopting very precisely specified standard operating procedures. Many pilots initially opposed these. One highly respected pilot, Captain David Davies, a senior test pilot, wrote a well-argued condemnation of standard operating procedures. Among other problems he suggested that they prevented pilots from thinking for themselves. Other senior pilots suggested that standard procedures would not fit all operational situations.

The chief pilot of one airline that had already adopted standard operating procedures suggested that Captain Davies should come and sit in the cockpit of some of their flights to observe their standard operating procedures in use in operational conditions. He did this and then flew with an airline that had not adopted standard operating procedures.

At the end of these observations Captain Davies had been completely persuaded of the benefits of standard operating procedures. He wrote 'I must admit my error and do a *volte face*. The only system that can survive is one that spells out in detail all operating procedures and insists on their application through a very high level of personal and crew discipline.'

Today, airline pilots accept the need for standard operating procedures and compliance is high. Occasionally, abnormal operating conditions in the operational environment mean that the standard operating procedure is inappropriate. In such cases the team leader should announce why and how a non-standard procedure is to be used. However, an unannounced departure from a standard operating procedure often signifies an error and should be challenged.

Creating a 'less steep' hierarchy

Other accidents revealed a problem that had not previously been fully accepted. The steepness of the professional hierarchy (where the captain was not open to input from the co-pilot) was a major problem. Cockpit voice recordings of various air disasters tragically revealed that co-pilots and flight engineers had attempted to bring critical information to the captain's attention in an unassertive way.

The enormous disaster at Tenerife Airport on 27 March 1977 was a terrible example of this. A total of 583 people burnt to death when two Jumbo jets collided on the runway. The cause of the accident was instantly apparent: the most senior and most highly respected pilot in the airline, who had a totally unblemished career record, had attempted to take off from a fog-shrouded runway without permission. His co-pilot and the flight engineer were heard on the cockpit voice recorder clearly telling the captain that permission had not been granted and that there was another aircraft on the runway. The captain brushed aside this input from his subordinates.

In the 1980s, in response to Tenerife and other accidents, airlines started setting up crew resource management (CRM) training programmes. CRM training includes a wide range of knowledge, skills, and attitudes including communications, situational awareness, problem solving, decision-making, and teamwork. It can be thought of as a management system that makes optimum use of all available resources—equipment, procedures, and people—to promote safety and enhance the efficiency of flight operations.

One of the principal vehicles of instruction on CRM courses is the use of appropriately instructive accident case studies, often illustrated with a video reconstruction.

The failure of co-pilots to speak up was addressed in the following way. During CRM courses, a series of accident case studies where co-pilots did not speak up was discussed. The senior pilots were asked by the trainer if there should be a formal policy, requirement, or procedure for juniors to speak up. Initially some of the senior pilots were reluctant, suggesting that co-pilots would often intervene inappropriately because of their inexperience.

The trainer then asked if the senior pilots would want their juniors to speak up if they really had made a mistake. A few senior pilots were still reluctant to admit that they would make such serious mistakes and refused to consider any formal speaking up policy. Happily, other senior pilots present on the courses managed to persuade the few to be more candid and accept that everyone makes mistakes from time to time. After further discussion the requirement for juniors to speak up was accepted.

However, some senior pilots worried that the 'cultural pendulum' might swing too far and a steep hierarchy would be replaced by a flat hierarchy. They feared that if junior pilots were encouraged to be more assertive they would have no respect for the experience of the senior pilots. These fears turned out to be completely unfounded. In a healthy professional culture there is always respect for experience.

CRM training helped to create a strong safety culture with a work force well informed about human error and high reliability issues. When new standard operating procedures were introduced as a result of lessons learned from incidents, personnel adopted them immediately as they could understand the reasons behind their introduction.

The lubricant of this new professional culture was candour. Both seniors and juniors could admit that they did not know something, had made an error, or had forgotten to do something that they ought to have done.

Using simulators to develop teamwork skills

A seminal piece of research was carried out by NASA. We think of NASA as being wholly interested with space, but its remit also includes aviation research. Furthermore, it also has close links with academia.

In the mid-1980s NASA borrowed 20 very experienced airline crews from a major American airline and put them in a high fidelity flight simulator. They videotaped the crews' performance for subsequent detailed analysis.

Each crew was asked to fly a simulated night flight from San Francisco to New York. About an hour into the 'flight', the experimenters created a 'simulated' fire in one of the aircraft's engines. The consequent failure of that engine's electrical generator then interacted with an undetected fault in the aircraft's emergency electrical switching system. As a result of this most of the aircraft's electrical power was lost at the same time.

This was a moderately severe problem to deal with. The crew, sitting in a semi-darkened cockpit, had to carry out the 'Engine Fire' checklist followed by the 'Loss of All Generators' checklist. This should have taken 2 or 3 minutes at most. They should then have turned the aircraft back to San Francisco and landed there. They needed to bear in mind that the aircraft would have trouble maintaining altitude over the Rocky Mountains having lost an engine and that a large amount of fuel would have to be dumped if they were land at a weight below the aircraft's 'maximum landing weight'.

As all of the crews were highly experienced, NASA and the pilots' own employers believed that the crews would all deal with this crisis reasonably well.

The observers were in for a big shock. The performance of most of the (highly experienced) crews in dealing with the simulated crisis was not very good. Their teamwork was a shambles.

Most of the crews took far longer to complete the checklists than was expected. Activity in some of the cockpits was described as 'mayhem'.

In most cases the captain physically took control of the aircraft while also simultaneously trying to troubleshoot the problems. He then gave instructions to the flight engineer. In many cases he overloaded the flight engineer with tasks, not necessarily in an appropriate order given their relative importance.

On many occasions the captains interrupted the flight engineers with less important matters. In one case the flight engineer was not allowed to complete any task before he was interrupted with another. The co-pilot was left out of the loop most of the time.

In contrast, with two of the 20 crews the captain recognized that this was a situation where he had to manage and to use all of the resources available to him. He handed over control of the flying of the aircraft to the co-pilot and asked him to get air traffic control to arrange the most expeditious route back to San Francisco avoiding the high terrain. He delegated the carrying out of the checklists to the flight engineer.

The captain then was able to 'sit back' and take an overview of the situation. He ensured that the checklists were completed correctly in a timely manner and communicated so that everyone was kept in the loop.

(Interestingly this is what happened in the British Airways Boeing 777 emergency landing in January 2008—the co-pilot landed the aircraft while the captain checked all the cockpit switches to try to troubleshoot why both engines seemed to have failed. The result was that not a single life was lost.)

> The industry saw a new vision of how the cockpit should be managed. There was more to being a good team leader than merely being a 'good operator' (aeroplane handler). The captain should be a team leader who had to communicate and manage the resources available to him.

Thus the emphasis was no longer exclusively on training the pilot to achieve excellence in flying the aeroplane. Instead he merely had to be a reasonably good aeroplane operator *and* at the same time a reasonably good team leader.

In many high reliability organizations teamwork training now takes place with high-fidelity simulators. Most people are not very good the first time they have to handle a crisis in a simulator. Doctors who have used medical simulators have found this.

Medical simulators use a realistic dummy, which can replicate a range of medical conditions. Actors can be used to play patient and staff roles in an 'operating theatre', 'anaesthetic room', 'ITU', 'A&E', and 'ward' based settings. The simulation can be video recorded so that the candidates can view and comment on their performance. This can be an uncomfortable experience at first ('did I really fail to check the patient's airway?').

Following this, a facilitated de-briefing session allows candidates the opportunity to learn through reflection, mutual support, and shared skills.

Simulators allow clinical teams to rehearse events that are rarely seen in everyday practice, such as anaphylaxis. It is often possible to induce for training purposes a 'mind lock', fixation situation where the trainee develops a flawed mental model and fails to appreciate that his actions, based on a flawed mental model, are not solving the problem.

After a small number of training sessions in the simulator almost all trainees are able to achieve a good standard of both technical and team skills.

Acceptance of auditing

No one likes to be watched doing their job. One gets neck ache looking over one's shoulder. But monitoring can be beneficial.

Pilots have now been persuaded to accept various systems to monitor how they operate the aircraft. One system monitors large amounts of data about how the aircraft is being flown. The data are collected from the aircraft's flight data recorders and analysed to find 'events' where the pilot's actions lay outside a range of safe flight parameters. The pilot will then receive a letter from his company within a few days of an interesting 'event' asking him to clarify exactly why he carried out a particular manoeuvre.

Pilots are not disciplined over events that are revealed solely through the use of the flight data monitoring system, although if there is an incident where there is damage to an aircraft then data from the monitoring system might be used to assist in the investigation.

The following scenario used to occur quite frequently. The presence of another aircraft beneath the flight path would lead air traffic control to refuse permission for a timely descent towards the destination airfield. When, eventually, the conflicting aircraft moved out of the way, descent was then authorized. However, by this time the aircraft was too far above the normal vertical profile to fly directly to the runway. Making the decent angle steeper to compensate would inevitably cause the aircraft's speed to increase and might result in the aircraft crossing the runway threshold at an excessive speed. Stopping the aircraft on the runway was then problematic.

Air traffic control would therefore offer the pilot of any aircraft that they had placed in such a 'too high' situation a longer, more circuitous route to the runway to 'get the height off'. However, such is the latent machismo of some pilots they sometimes saw such a situation as a challenge and they would still try to make a straight in approach ('there I was at 12 000ft and only 30 miles from the runway and I still got in'). This could all be quite exciting but occasionally produced disappointing results!

As a result of the monitoring systems, pilots now feel less disposed to taking such risks. Flying is certainly duller than it once was but the incident and accident rate has been substantially reduced.

Applying such ideas in healthcare

Doctors might be appalled that these ideas could be applied in healthcare.

However, consider this. When we settle back into seat 6B for our flight to Toulouse with our children sitting on either side of us, are we reassured that the pilots will be following precisely specified standard operating procedures and using pre-take-off checklists? When we get to Toulouse, is it a good thing that the pilot probably will not attempt an exciting steep approach, but instead will follow the rules?

When the pilot or his loved ones are placed on our operating table should we not have a high reliability service to offer him in return? Is it not right to use standard operating procedures, such as checklists, to ensure that he receives appropriate thromboprophylaxis and antibiotic prophylaxis, and that he gets the right operation on the correct side? Should we not try to adopt less steep hierarchies? Would regular monitoring of our activity - with positive feedback to enhance performance - not be a good idea?

Martin Bromiley, an airline pilot and the husband of Elaine Bromiley, to whom this book is dedicated, did expect that the healthcare professionals treating his wife would operate in a safety culture equivalent to the one in which he operates.

Sadly, we let him down in the worst way possible.

Team resource management/non-technical skills

During the process to improve teamwork in the aviation and nuclear power industries it has been felt necessary to give names to the types of behaviours that have been observed to enhance good teamwork. At the same time it is also thought to be important to label behaviours that inhibit good teamwork.

Videos have been produced of good teamwork in a simulator and also of poor teamwork. Trainers and managers have watched these videos and have agreed on standard terms for the behaviours observed. One might imagine that it would be difficult to achieve consensus in such a subjective task. However, after a series of videos were studied and discussed, the observers found it easier to be consistent with labelling the behaviours observed.

From this work some high reliability industries have developed a system of desired 'non-technical skills' sets that teams and team leaders should possess.

The team leader has to achieve an appropriate balance between the leading the team and listening to their input while at the same time ensuring high situation awareness in the team.

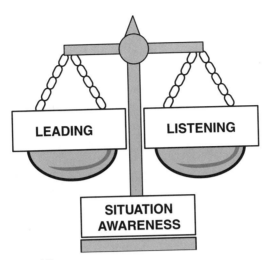

Fig. 8.1 Team leader skills.

The team leader must provide clear leadership for the team while being receptive to team suggestions. The team leader must state his opinion but allow team members to assert their views. Every one in the team should be 'appropriately assertive'. The team leader should recognize that aggressive behaviours on his part or from senior colleagues will induce passive behaviours in junior colleagues. While such a situation might seem expedient at any given time, in the long term the team will lose valuable input from front-line junior personnel.

Let us look at the following three principal elements in turn:

♦ leadership/managerial skills

♦ co-operation/communication

♦ situation awareness.

Leadership/managerial skills

Getting the job done to the highest standard

Effective leadership and managerial skills result in the successful completion of the task by the motivated, fully functioning team through co-ordination, persuasion, and discipline.

The core of effective leadership is to set the highest priority on the completion of a given task to the highest possible standard. Leadership responsibilities include the active and goal-directed co-ordination of the working activities within the team. This is always a reciprocal process. Without complementary behaviour by the team, leadership behaviour is less effective. All team members are expected to dedicate their efforts and initiative to the safe and efficient achievement of the team goals. Team responsibilities include monitoring and challenging each other whenever differences in concepts or actions are perceived.

The team leader should be a person whose ideas and actions influence the thought and the behaviour of others. Through the use of example and persuasion, and an understanding of the goals and desires of the group, the leader becomes a means of change and influence. It is important to distinguish between (1) leadership, which is acquired, and (2) authority, which is assigned. Leadership is one aspect of teamwork, and the success of a leader depends on the quality of his/her relationship in the team.

The team leader should provide general standards and directions for the completion of the different tasks. The tasks are allocated according to defined roles, competence, specific experience, as well as to the present level of workload of the team members.

Interactive briefings should be carried out before safety-critical operations commence and during the procedure the team leader is always open for the contributions from other team members. A leader motivates, activates, and monitors others and encourages the team to monitor and challenge him and each other in a constructive way.

In a high reliability culture, the team also looks to the future and ensures that the causes of failures (equipment, systems, and procedures), human errors, and inadequacies in training programmes are addressed in order to make the operation safer next time.

Elements of leadership and managerial skills

- *Use of authority and assertiveness*. The team leader has to achieve a fine balance between asserting his authority and allowing an appropriate level of team member participation. If the situation requires, decisive actions are expected.

- *Providing and maintaining standards*. The team leader's prime role is to create a disciplined atmosphere where activities are carried out to a high professional standard. The compliance with standard procedures for the task completion should be ensured. Therefore, the team should mutually supervise and intervene in case of any deviations from the standard. In abnormal conditions, it might be necessary to apply non-standard procedures. Such deviations should be announced and agreed by the team.

- *Planning and co-ordination.* In order to achieve high performance and to prevent workload peaks or dips, organized task sharing and delegation has to be established. Plans and intentions have to be communicated so that the whole team understands the goals and activities of the team. Team leaders should ensure that team members work only in areas in which they are competent.

- *Workload management.* This requires clear prioritization of primary and secondary operational tasks. Based on sound planning, tasks are distributed appropriately among the team. Interruptions can induce errors and should be avoided. Signs of stress and fatigue are communicated and taken into account as factors affecting performance.

- *Delegation and off-loading.* When in threatening or difficult situations, many team leaders experience the natural urge to 'take control' of tasks from their (usually) less experienced colleagues. This may be counterproductive in situations where critical demands exceed the capacity for a single person to do everything alone. The team leader can become overloaded, thus unable to maintain 'situation awareness' and to direct the team members efficiently. 'Off-loading' is the difficult practice of delegating responsibility for tasks to team members, even if they might perform these tasks slightly less efficiently than the team leader, allowing the team leader to 'step back' and manage the whole operation.

- *Error management and system improvement.* Errors by team members should be handled appropriately without unjust blame. The team leader can create a candid atmosphere by describing his own errors. There should be awareness of previous adverse event scenarios. It is the responsibility of everyone in the system to consider how improvements can be made, both to personal competence and to the 'system' as a whole. It is the team leader's responsibility to ensure that critical incident reports are completed if appropriate. The team leader must challenge any perception within the team that error-inducing situations cannot be changed.

This last point contrasts with the 'culture of low expectations' often found in healthcare.

Co-operation/communication

Winning their hearts and minds

This element includes those team behaviours that build co-operation and trust within the team. All members of the team should feel that their input is valued. Communications within the team should allow the effective transfer of information, ideas, and emotions.

The team members should feel that they are an integral part of a well-run, well-organized operation in which their inputs are essential to reach the commonly valued goals and the overall success of the operation. Complete candour within the team is absolutely essential.

In an operating theatre a junior theatre nurse may not be able to offer detailed surgical input to the consultant, but could be asked to confirm if the procedure is being initiated on the correct side.

Co-operation requires *team building and maintenance*, so that co-operative actions are based on a mutual agreement of team members in a positive group climate. Such a climate is also obtained by factors such as *consideration/support of other team members* and *conflict-solving skills*. Co-operation deals with the question of how people function as a working group. It does not refer to the quality or quantity of the work itself.

In order to ensure proper support and the participation from all parts of the team, active care is taken to establish and maintain communication. Subscribers to the 'old school' of leadership might question the importance of communicating **emotions** as stated in the summary above. However, team members should be able to communicate their unease if they perceive there is a problem that is not being properly handled. Good co-operation is largely dependent on open and candid communication between team members.

Elements of co-operation

The summary definition of co-operation comprises different elements.

- *Team building and maintenance.* Establishing positive and candid interpersonal relations and active participation of team members in fulfilling tasks.

- *Consideration of others.* Acceptance of others and understanding their personal condition.

- *Support of others.* Giving help to other team members in case they need assistance.

- *Solving interpersonal conflicts.* Articulation of different interpersonal positions with suggestions for solutions.

Elements of communication

Effective communication comprises different elements:

- *Clearly stating the 'need' or the intention of the message.* Providing sufficient background information so that the purpose of the communication cannot be misunderstood.

- *Clearly imparting the basic message.* Using appropriate terminology and avoiding verbal short-cuts (pronouns, abbreviations, etc.). Stating the obvious to ensure all elements of the message are conveyed.
- *Ensuring comprehension of the message.* Expecting and giving read-back.
- *Awareness of 'tone' and non-verbal communication.* Considering the emotional implications of the way the message is passed. An atmosphere should be created where a team member is able to communicate his/her unease effectively.
- *Appreciation of the receiver's situation.* Considering the most appropriate medium and timing for a message (e.g. avoiding making a telephone call to someone in order to pass a non-urgent message at a time when it might interrupt their work). Does the receiver have the technical knowledge to understand my message?

Situation awareness

Not missing that vital detail

Team situation awareness is the function of ensuring that each member of the team is able to create a mental model, appropriate to their work role, which accurately reflects the exact state of all the relevant variables in the operational situation over which they are expected to exercise control.

The creation and maintenance of situation awareness within a team requires formalized processes. The system must ensure that the team is provided with all the necessary information (in healthcare this would be the patient's notes, test results, etc.) and the team must check that this is available. Clinicians must examine the patient appropriately, monitoring and reporting changes in the patient's condition. They must keep complete, legible, and accurate patient records. They must also be aware of the availability and serviceability of all equipment that is to be used during the procedure.

The team leader should be aware of the experience level of each of the members of the team and the limitations on their areas of competence. The team leader should also be aware if any members of the team are stressed, tired, or unwell.

The team must ensure that everyone feels able to offer input on their perception of the situation. The possibility of problems or error must be considered. It might be necessary to explicitly discuss likely threats.

References

1 *The Inquiry into the management of the care of children receiving complex heart surgery at the Bristol Royal Infirmary* (chaired by Professor Ian Kennedy) Final Report Command Paper: CM 5207. Also available at: http://www.bristol-inquiry.org.uk/ (accessed 12 October 2008).

2 **Quine L.** Workplace bullying in NHS community trust: staff questionnaire survey. *Br Med J* 1999; **318**: 228–32.

Chapter 9

When carers deliberately cause harm

Abuse can occur in situations where one party is unable to take care of themselves or protect themselves from harm or exploitation. Healthcare workers must be alert and able to identify markers and signs of abuse in vulnerable patients of all ages, and every healthcare organization should have an appropriate leader(s) to oversee the protection of vulnerable individuals.

Sadly, abuse does occur at the hands of professional carers and healthcare workers. It is often unrecognized over a long period of time perhaps because of denial by fellow workers. Delivery of healthcare demands a high level of trust between the deliverers of care and between carers and their patients. Abusive and criminal behaviour is often met with incredulity because it challenges the principles of how we work.

The issues of child protection and the care of vulnerable adults lies beyond the remit of this book but the following case study may serve as a reminder that when there is no other rational explanation you must be prepared to think the unthinkable in order to protect patients.

In February 2004 a 41-year-old man was admitted to the emergency department of the Horton Hospital in Oxfordshire complaining of abdominal pain and vomiting. He was seen promptly by a junior doctor who felt the most likely diagnosis was alcohol withdrawal and gastritis. On admission his blood glucose was 6.4 mmol/l but 2 hours later the patient was agitated and rapidly became unconscious and had a seizure. The blood glucose was now found to be 1.6 mmol/l. After administration of intravenous dextrose the patient made a full recovery and went home a few days later. The consultant in charge of the case wrote in the notes 'it is difficult to explain the sequence of events' and he filed a report with clinical risk management. Later he was discussing the events with colleagues when it became apparent that they too had seen cases where they harboured doubts about exactly what had happened. A review of records identified 10 cases in the preceding 2 months where patients had rapidly deteriorated in the emergency department. Reluctantly, foul play was suspected. A check of rotas for all emergency department staff identified one individual who had been on duty for all 10 cases. After a long and detailed investigation, nurse Ben Geen was subsequently found guilty of two charges of murder and 15 counts of grievous bodily harm.

Readers may be aware of other UK cases–Dr Harold Shipman, Beverley Allitt, and Colin Norris. A recent study of cases from around the world[1] identified 90 criminal prosecutions of healthcare workers between 1970 and 2006 for serial murder of patients. Fifty-four were convicted and 24 were still unresolved. In total, 2113 suspicious patient deaths were attributed to the 54 convicted individuals.

Some common threads appear to run through many of these cases. Bruce Sackman was an investigator on the team that brought nurse Kristen Gilbert to trial for murdering four patients and attempting to murder three more and he described so-called 'red flags' that should signal suspicion (quoted by Pyrek[2]). These include the following:

- The subject predicts the patient's demise.
- Staff and family have not foreseen the patient's death.
- There are no eye witnesses to the event.
- The subject is seen with the patient immediately before the agonal event.
- A limited range of potentially lethal but readily available drugs is employed (insulin, potassium, opioids, muscle relaxants, adrenaline (epinephrine), and lidocaine). These are not routinely looked for at autopsy.
- Record keeping may be incomplete or crucial results missing from the record.
- The subject often appears superficially personable but may have difficulties in relationships.
- There may have been problems in past educational or work records.
- Staff give the subject a nickname before suspicions are aroused (colleagues referred to Geen as 'Ben Allitt' because he always seemed to be around when patients rapidly deteriorated).
- Killing is non-confrontational.
- The subject insists the patient died of natural causes.
- The subject shows no remorse.

- The subject craves notoriety or wants to be centre stage. They are calm under questioning.
- The subject may kill or attempt to kill when off duty as well as on duty.

Human factors experts have a term for cases such as these: Intentional (or deliberate) Adverse Events. Fortunately they are extremely rare events. However, when they do occur they are almost always disproportionately more destructive than accidental adverse events. The perpetrator often goes to great lengths to avoid discovery and to maximize the harm.

Nor is this a problem unique to healthcare. A handful of intentional adverse events are believed to have occurred in other safety critical domains. In four or five air accidents (and we exclude here the events of 9/11/2001) the pilot was suspected of crashing his aircraft deliberately, killing all his passengers in the process. Investigations subsequently revealed significant problems in his mental state or private life.

One might cling to the belief that a case like Shipman would not recur because the publicity creates a level of awareness that would prevent a repetition. Alas this might not always be the case. In many industries we have seen a widely publicized adverse event being repeated with an almost identical scenario not long afterwards, even though people thought surely it could not happen again.

Without the systematic adoption of appropriate formal preventive measures a repetition is possible. On 12 February 2009 BBC Radio 4 broadcast a program entitled: "Could Shipman Happen Again?" On the program Dame Janet Smith, who chaired the Harold Shipman Inquiry, criticized the system of death certification in England and Wales. She said that progress in implementing the recommendations in her report has been slow.

None of the High Reliability Organizations currently has any system in place to specifically target intentional adverse events. Healthcare might even be in a position to take the lead in this hitherto neglected and acute area of risk management. The use of 'red flag' recognition, the filing of a critical incident report, and communicating with colleagues as encouraged in a progressive safety culture may assist in detection. Fortunately this hastened the detection of Ben Geen's activities.

References

1 Yorker BC, Kizer KW, Lampe P, Forrest ARW, Lannan JM, Russell DA. Serial murder by healthcare professionals. *J Forensic Sci* 2006; **51**: 1362–71.
2 Pyrek KM. Healthcare serial killers: recognizing the red flags. *Forensic Nurse* Online. 20 April 2005. http://www.forensicnursemag.com/.

Chapter 10

Patient safety toolbox

Practical ways to enhance the safety of your patients

Safer clinical communications

The first and most effective action that you can take immediately to enhance your patient's safety is to attempt to achieve the highest standard in your safety-critical clinical, verbal, and written communications.

As we have seen, a significant proportion of the adverse events described in this book involved a maddeningly avoidable misunderstanding. Research shows that these communication errors are 'twice as frequent as errors due to inadequate clinical skill'.

It is interesting to remember that doctors spend hours studying rare medical conditions which they might encounter only once or twice in their whole career. On the other hand the evidence is that, on average, every few days a hospital doctor will encounter a patient whose medical condition is being or has been significantly compromised as a consequence of a miscommunication between clinicians. Until now there has been little awareness of this critical issue, and little has been done to address it.

We believe that it would be wise to invest time studying the causes of communication failures as described in Chapter 6. You should consider adopting some of the safe communication behaviours that have been shown to work successfully in a number of safety critical domains.

Safer patient notes

Another area where an instant improvement to patient safety could be made is with respect to the 'reliability' of your patient's notes. You should take 'lead responsibility' for the notes of any patient who comes into your care even temporarily.

Write clearly, using capital letters if necessary. Print your name and leave a contact number. Better still, obtain and use a self-inking rubber stamp with your name and contact number.

Get into the habit of writing an up to date summary of the case in the current notes. It is extremely important for handover, it makes you focus on the current problems, and it ensures that important information and recent investigations are readily available. If necessary, re-sort the notes into a logical sequence. Remember the lesson of case 5 (p93). Should important warnings be visible on both the outside and the inside of the notes? (Case 14, p107) Draw attention to the existence of other sets of notes for the same patient. 'Cleanse' the notes of other patient's results and incorrect addressogram labels. All these actions may take a little extra time but not only will they enhance patient safety, they will make the process of care more efficient - for both yourself and your colleagues. This will be because there will be less wasted effort searching for information.

Keep a small notebook. When you order a test for a patient, write it in the notebook. Cross the entry off when the test comes back. If the patient moves on to another department it is your responsibility to ensure the test result follows the patient. Take 'lead responsibility' for any test you order.

Awareness of patient safety issues in your specialty or department

In recent years there have been over a dozen cases in the U.K. where vincristine has been administered intrathecally with fatal results (of which cases 6, 7 and 8 were examples, see p94–100). These cases reflected a systemic failure of healthcare to learn the lessons of past accidents. Other 'threats' include the similarities in medication packaging which creates a continuing hazard in many specialties (p42–43)

One might have thought that some patient safety hazards ought to be very obvious. However we see cases where even experienced clinicians seem to have been quite unaware of what would seem to be obvious risks. This was the case with the danger of using dry swabs with diathermy (pages 49 and 249).

Thus it is important that you should actively develop an awareness of the patient safety hazards in your specialty or department. What errors or error-inducing situations keep on occurring? Use the internet to search for errors that have happened in similar circumstances. Regularly visit patient safety websites such as www.npsa.org

Check the notice-boards and documentation in your department. Is all of the necessary information (such as treatment protocols) readily available (case 12, p103)? Are new personnel safely inducted into your department? Do they know how to arrange investigations (p164)?

Improve patient safety in the future

You must use your Trust's critical incident reporting system to report any incidents or error-inducing situations that you encounter. This will improve healthcare in the future.

You could organise short, regular patient safety courses or meetings for your department. The format should generally follow the sequence in this book: show delegates the evidence that there is a problem, show them that successful, workable solutions are available. Create presentations of instructive case studies. Facilitate a discussion about practical measures that can address these issues.

Be assertive in advancing patient safety

You will note that many of the measures that we suggest involve taking 'lead responsibility' for various patient safety activities. It is easier to do this if you are able to display assertiveness appropriately. High reliability organizations have learned the hard way that it is essential that all their personnel should be assertive. This does not mean being aggressive or rude. You can be both assertive and tactful.

Personnel in some high reliability organizations are given the following bill of rights:

♦ You have the right to have and express your own ideas and feelings.
♦ You have the right to be treated with respect.
♦ You have the right to ask for information from others, and the right to be able to say that you are unaware of something or do not understand something.
♦ You have the right to change your mind
♦ You have the right to make mistakes.
♦ You have the right to make decisions or statements without having to apologize for them.
♦ You have the right to feel and express emotions, both positive and negative, without feeling that it is weak or undesirable to do so.
♦ You have the right to refuse demands on you.
♦ You have the right to judge yourself and your own actions. You must be prepared to bear the consequences.

Think infection control

Wash your hands between every patient contact (and encourage your whole team to do the same).

Prescribe antibiotics appropriately avoiding prolonged courses if possible.

Ensure antibiotic prophylaxis and thromboprophylaxis is given (in the context of surgical procedures use a checklist to help ensure compliance).

And finally (really!)

- *Remember*—adopting the techniques we have described is not going to be easy.
- It is very likely that other doctors and nurses may think that you are odd when you first start to use them.
- You may even be ridiculed.
- You will need courage.
- But persevere and you ***will*** be a safer doctor.
- You will also improve your efficiency. Following these procedures will mean you will spend less time chasing missing test results, etc.

References

1   Parker J, Coiera E. Improving clinical communication: a view from psychology. *J Am Med Informatics Assoc* 2000; 7: 453–61.

Chapter 11

Conclusions

In our rush to embrace the great technological advances that have occurred in medicine over the last 50 years (mass immunization, great advances in imaging technology, laparoscopic surgery, the promise of diagnostic and treatment advances from sequencing the human genome to name but a few), the attention of the medical profession has been diverted from the problem of human error in healthcare. When an airliner or train crashes, the enormity of the event is apparent for all to see. The fact that medical accidents happen to individual patients in individual hospitals makes them much less visible than accidents in other safety-critical industries. This has been a major factor in hiding the scale of the problem of medical error and thus in perpetuating it. However, times are changing and the public, through the media, are becoming increasingly aware that error in healthcare exists and that it is a major problem.

It goes without saying that the principal victims of human error are those patients (and their loved ones) who suffer harm as a result of their carers' well intentioned, but flawed care. However, there are other victims. As a consequence of this systemic neglect of patient safety issues, doctors and nurses work in an environment where they are often 'set up' to be the final, all too visible link in an error chain (what Americans would call a 'patsy'). These doctors and nurses are the second victims of error. The burden that many must carry, knowing that they have harmed a patient, can have a profound effect. The burden of error extends still further—to the tax-payer. This is a hidden cost, but it is enormous. Millions of pounds in extra treatment are required to rectify the effects of error, many extra bed days are wasted and, for some, ongoing disability requires additional resources. Thus if we, as a profession, can make a concerted effort to reduce healthcare-associated error, everyone is a winner.

While individual clinicians aim for excellence in their clinical skills, little concerted effort is applied to help doctors learn how to communicate more safely, how to carry out safety-critical checks using checklists or how to work within the framework of a team. Without good teamwork skills a significant proportion of the day-to-day efforts of the expert clinician may be wasted. A surgeon may perform the most brilliant colectomy for bowel cancer, achieving complete cancer clearance with the prospect of genuine cure. However, all will be in vain if he and his team forget to give the patient appropriate thrombo-prophylaxis and as a consequence the patient drops dead from a massive pulmonary embolus 10 days after the operation. So, clearly, the performance of the team is critical to the successful outcome of any treatment.

The high reliability organizations that we have described in this book have been able to transform their safety record despite working in hazardous environments. Their road to safety has not been an easy one and in many cases they have learnt the hard way—from their *own* experiences rather than from those of others. The systems they have developed are remarkably similar to each other and they centre principally around regular training of their workforce in the concept of human error and in simple techniques that can be used to prevent or mitigate the effects of error. As a consequence not a single life has been lost on board a British jet airliner in the last 20 years.

We have tried in this book to help the reader understand that clinical error is common, that there are common themes leading to error, and that high reliability organizations have been able to improve their safety record by attention to human factors training of their personnel. We have tried also to demonstrate that the same techniques that are used to reduce error in high reliability organizations can be directly applied to the healthcare setting.

We have already said that healthcare differs in several important aspects from flying aircraft, not least because patients are often very sick and therefore vulnerable and because the 'operations' of healthcare organizations are enormously diverse. Healthcare organizations have the added problem over high reliability organizations that the number of staff to be trained in safety techniques is so large. An airline has far fewer staff to train relative to passenger numbers.

However, we believe that there are more similarities than differences between the experiences of error in high reliability organizations and errors that occur in healthcare.

We know also that the concepts and practical advice that we have outlined in this book are not the sole solution to error in healthcare and we are not for one moment suggesting that error will disappear overnight as long as the reader reads this book and adheres to the advice therein. Error reduction requires many things (principally, from the individual's perspective, a change of attitude and an understanding of error reduction techniques). Reading a book is not enough, just as attending a single patient safety course and ticking the 'attended' box is not enough eiher. However, it is a start on the *continuous* journey of patient safety training.

We know that doctors and nurses who become disciples of safety after they have read *Practical patient safety* will face scepticism from others, indeed even ridicule.

We know that the regularity with which safety checks must be done can be boring. If wrong site surgery occurs roughly once in every 15 000 operations, that is a lot of checklisting to do to avoid that one error. But what an error! What terrible implications! It is of course not difficult to see why so many healthcare workers would lapse in this checklisting process. But this under-sores why they need simple tools to prevent such errors.

Using a checklist is rather like putting on a seatbelt before a car journey. Those of us in our late forties or fifties can remember the time when people did not wear seatbelts. At that time many people saw the law requiring the use of seatbelts as a serious assault on their human rights. Others felt that the effort of putting the seatbelt on was excessive in view of the risk ('I'm only going down to the shops!').

In one way the latter group may be right if you look at the numbers. The chance of dying in a road traffic accident in a lifetime in the UK is roughly 1 in 200. To mitigate this risk, 199 other people will have to put on their seatbelts for every journey for the whole of their lives. This equates to a total of perhaps 50 000 'unnecessary' uses of the seatbelt in a lifetime for each these 199 people.

However, we now have a culture of seatbelt use. Few of us would stop wearing seatbelts if the law were repealed. Few can argue with the statement that wearing a seatbelt is the right thing to do. One day the medical profession will see the use of checklists as the right thing to do. We hope this little book will play some role in accelerating the process.

We have heard many doctors dismiss the concept of checklists, arguing that they are not necessary to prevent wrong site surgery, because 'we just wouldn't make that mistake'. The pilot, on the other hand, who will fly you to your holiday destination this year or to your international medical conference has no problem with the mundane process of checklisting. He or she is a highly trained, highly skilled professional, but he or she is also sensible enough to know that even the very best pilots and the very best crews can, from time to time, make an error. They know that without using checklists they put not only the lives of their passengers at risk, but also the lives of their crew and indeed themselves. And so when you next sit on a plane be reassured that the crew will *check* that the doors are closed. When you hear the captain say 'doors to cross-check', you will know you are in safe hands. It is probable of course that the crew wouldn't possibly forget to close the doors—and yet they keep on using those four words—'doors to cross-check'! We know why.

We are acutely aware that many of the healthcare workers with whom you will be working and communicating will not have read this book and they will not be familiar with the concepts and terminology that is used in it. We know also that some of the communication tools described may appear, at first sight, to be facile, bizarre, onerous, or socially awkward. Those 'safety-critical' industries that have adopted similar communication safety tools have shown that they can be 100% effective if used by both parties, but even if used by just one party to a conversation they can none the less enhance safety. So try not to feel too awkward when using them. Be reassured also that you will not be alone in using these safety tools. A growing number of progressive hospitals in the USA and Canada have decided that these tools can be adapted to the often exceptionally demanding requirements of healthcare and have started to use many of them.

Be brave! The fact that you have at least bought this book means you are in the vanguard of change.

Glossary

In the early 1990s a conference was held on the subject of airline safety. The delegate of one airline commented that it was having occasional problems because its pilots were making a particular type of mistake with a new piece of equipment. The representative of another airline commented that they were having the same problem but they had given it a different name.

It was soon realized that the problem might have been somewhat more widespread than had been appreciated. Owing to non-standardized terminology it was not appearing in the incident databases to its true extent.

The first step in successfully addressing human error issues in an organization or even an entire industry is to ensure that everyone speaks a common language. If there is an understanding of basic risk management concepts, well-informed and precise discussions involving all ranks of personnel can take place.

You will probably want to improve your healthcare system by making critical incident reports about systemic failures. Using the correct human factors terminology may make it more likely that hospital authorities will take remedial action. Here is glossary of useful patient safety/human factors terminology.

Accident An adverse event following a combination of human errors, system failures, and a chance event.

ACRM anaesthetic crisis resource management See CRM.

Active errors/active failures (concept contrasts with latent or system failures) Errors and violations committed at the 'sharp end' of the system—by pilots, air traffic controllers, doctors, nurses, ships' crews, control room operators, maintenance personnel, and the like. Such unsafe acts are likely to have a direct impact on the safety of the system. Because of the immediacy of their adverse effects, these acts are termed active failures.

Adverse event Any injury caused by medical care. Examples include:

+ pneumothorax from central venous catheter placement
+ anaphylaxis to intravenous penicillin
+ postoperative wound infection
+ hospital-acquired infection
+ surgical procedure carried out on the wrong patient.

Identifying an incident as an adverse event does not imply 'error,' 'negligence', or poor quality care. It simply indicates that an undesirable clinical outcome resulted from some aspect of diagnosis or therapy and not the underlying disease process. Thus, pneumothorax from central venous catheter placement counts as an adverse event regardless of insertion technique. Similarly, postoperative wound infections count as adverse events even if the operation proceeded with optimal adherence to sterile procedures, the patient received appropriate antibiotic prophylaxis in the peri-operative setting, and so on.

However, some adverse events are the result of avoidable human errors and teamwork failures.

Adverse drug event (ADE) An adverse event involving medication use. Examples include:

◆ anaphylaxis to penicillin
◆ heparin-induced thrombocytopenia
◆ aminoglycoside-induced renal failure, ototoxicity, and vestibulopathy
◆ agranulocytosis from chloramphenicol
◆ error by clinician—wrong dose, wrong route, etc.

As with the more general term, adverse event, there is no necessary relation to error or poor quality of care. In other words, ADEs include expected adverse drug reactions (or 'side-effects') as well as events due to error. Thus, a serious allergic reaction to penicillin in a patient with no such previous history is an ADE, but so is the same reaction in a patient who does have a known allergy history but receives penicillin due to a prescribing oversight. Ignoring the distinction between expected medication side-effects and ADEs due to errors may seem misleading, but a similar distinction can be achieved with the concept of preventability. All ADEs due to error are preventable, but other ADEs not warranting the label 'error' may also be preventable.

Alert phrase A predetermined phrase that an operator can utter to draw other team members' attention to uncertainty, departures from normal or safe procedures, or other situations that may represent evidence of an incipient adverse event.

Ambiguity This is an unresolved/unexplained conflict or contradiction between two sets of information, instrument indications or a difference between what is happening and what was expected to happen. It may also be said to occur when someone does something that is not normal in the operational situation. Ambiguities are often the first signs of an incipient adverse event.

Anchoring error A cognitive bias in which past (especially recent) cases are allowed to bias current diagnostic evaluation. An example might be a physician who saw two recent cases presenting with a certain set of symptoms and signs that proved to have polymyalgia rheumatica, now assuming that subsequent patients with similar presentations have the same disease, thereby discounting other diagnostic possibilities.

Assertiveness training Assertiveness is the antidote to the passivity that is evident in junior team members in hierarchical organizations. As many major adverse events could have been prevented if juniors had been more assertive, assertiveness training is now provided in many organizations.

Attitude The tendency to react favourably or unfavourably towards certain stimuli, such as individuals, groups of people, practices, customs, and institutions. An example might be the subject's attitude toward carrying out formal verbalized checking procedures. Attitudes cannot be directly observed and have to be inferred by observing the subject's behaviour.

High reliability organizations have used attitude surveys to measure the effectiveness of their safety training programmes in modifying potentially hazardous employee attitudes.

Authority gradient The balance of decision-making power or the steepness of command hierarchy in a team. Members of a team with a domineering, overbearing, or dictatorial team leader experience a steep authority gradient. Expressing concerns, questioning, or even simply clarifying instructions would require considerable determination on the part of team members who perceive their input as devalued or unwelcome. Most teams require some degree of authority gradient, otherwise roles are blurred and decisions cannot be made in a timely fashion.

Behaviour A subject's observable actions in the workplace. High reliability organizations observe the behaviour of employees to check that they are working safely.

Blame culture A culture that assumes that errors are moral failures. It is convenient for managers to blame front-line staff for accidents in order to distract attention from their poorly designed procedures and inadequate training courses.

Call-back American term for 'Read back' q.v.

Checklist The algorithmic listing of actions to be performed in a safety-critical situation. In healthcare Acute Cardiac Life Support (ACLS) protocols for treating cardiac arrest ensure that, no matter how often performed by a given practitioner, no step should be forgotten.

Close call (American term) An event or situation that did not produce patient injury, but only because of chance. This good fortune might reflect robustness of the patient (e.g. a patient with penicillin allergy receives penicillin, but has no reaction) or a fortuitous, timely intervention (e.g. a nurse happens to realize that a physician wrote an order in the wrong chart). Such events are termed 'near-miss' incidents in the UK.

CRM (crew resource management or crisis resource management) A range of approaches to ensure that a team is able to function effectively in normal and crisis situations by accessing all of the mental and physical resources of all of the members of the team. The term 'crew resource management' arose in aviation following analysis of the cockpit voice recordings of crashed aircraft. This revealed that the crew had had all the information they needed to sort out a problem but that the captain had failed to use all the resources available to him. In anaesthesia, some progressive training programmes are using simulators and use the term '(anaesthetic) crisis resource management' for this type of team training.

Culpability of errors Some errors are clearly more 'culpable' than others. Consider two cases:

1 A doctor who makes a 'slip of the tongue' when stressed during an acute event.

2 A doctor who is known to routinely consult without reading the patients' records, carries out inadequate examinations, and who then makes a wrong diagnosis.

The latter is clearly more culpable than the former.

Culture of low expectations The term 'a culture of low expectations' was devised by Mark Chassin and Elise Becher. When a system routinely produces error-inducing situations (missing paperwork, miscommunications between team members, changes of plan), clinicians become inured to malfunction. In such a system, events that should be regarded as Red Flags, as a major warning of impending danger are ignored as a *normal* operating conditions.

Error An error is defined as the failure of a planned action to be completed as intended (i.e. error of execution) or the use of a wrong plan to achieve an aim (i.e. an error of planning).

Error chain A term created by human factors trainers to describe the sequence of situations, events, and errors that leads to an accident. While accidents may seem inexorable, the 'chain' metaphor suggests the possibility of a 'weak link' where operators can intervene to 'break the chain'.

Facilitation (contrasts with didactic instruction) High reliability organizations have to modify the attitudes and behaviour of their personnel when these are shown to be hazardous. 'Facilitation' is a technique that helps personnel to develop attitudes and behaviours that are appropriate and effective when working in a team in safety-critical environments. Accident case studies are presented and the facilitator asks delegates to review their own attitudes and behaviours in the light of these cases and their own experiences.

Note: Instructing people to change their attitudes and behaviour normally has limited success.

Forcing function An aspect of a design that prevents a target action from being performed inappropriately. For example, automatic teller machines now do not issue the money until the bank card has been removed from the machine first. In the past when the sequence was the other way round many people collected their money but left their card in the machine. An important 'forcing function' introduced in healthcare is the placing of concentrated potassium chloride in locked cupboards.

Hierarchy The relationship between seniors and subordinates within an organization *as perceived by the subordinate*. It reflects the extent to which the less powerful members of the culture expect and accept that power is distributed unequally. In a 'steep hierarchy' there is considerable deference by subordinates to their superiors. Expressing concerns, questioning arrangements, or even clarifying instructions require considerable determination on the part of team members. The latter may perceive their input as devalued and unwelcome.

In a shallower hierarchy there is a general preference for consultation over prescriptive methods. Subordinates are comfortable in approaching, and if necessary, contradicting their superiors. It is important to note that hierarchies that are too shallow can produce a lack of discipline that can be as dangerous as a too steep hierarchy.

High reliability organizations (HROs) Organizations that, although operating with safety-critical technologies in dynamic and hazardous environments, manage to achieve very low rates of accidents. Their core philosophy is to expect and avoid failure rather than to achieve success.

Human factors An applied science 'concerned to optimize the relationship between people and their activities by the systematic application of the human sciences, integrated within the framework of systems engineering'. Initially developed to maximize production and profitability in the manufacturing industry, human factors science has been successfully developed and employed to manage human error in 'high-risk' domains.

Incident reporting Investigations of major accidents in a number of domains often reveal that similar events had nearly occurred previously but had been stopped but fortuitous circumstances. Incident reporting systems are designed to gather data on the latent or system failures that lead to 'near misses' and accidents. These data are used to redesign training programmes and standard operating procedures.

Intentional unsafe act A deliberate act of harm or damage by a psychopathic employee. Incidents have been reported in several safety-critical industries.

Lapse An error of memory (contrast with mistake, slip).

Latent failures/system failures (concept contrasts with active failures) Long-term situations that induce human error or inhibit error detection or prevention. These are usually associated with poor management.

Learning curve The acquisition of any new skill is associated with the potential for lower-than-expected success rates or higher-than-expected complication rates. This phenomenon is often known as a 'learning curve.' In some cases, this learning curve can be quantified in terms of the number of procedures that must be performed before an operator can replicate the outcomes of more experienced operators or teams. While learning curves are almost inevitable when new procedures emerge or new providers are in training, minimizing their impact is a patient safety imperative. One option is to perform initial operations or procedures under the supervision of more experienced operators. Surgical and procedural simulators may play an increasingly important part in decreasing the impact of learning curves on patients, by allowing acquisition of relevant skills in laboratory settings.

Mental models Mental models are psychological representations of real, hypothetical, or imaginary situations. Scottish psychologist Kenneth Craik (1943) first proposed mental models as the basis for anticipating events and explaining events.

Mind lock A term created by human factors trainers to describe a situation where a subject fails to change his mental model even when there is evidence that his interactions with the system he is attempting to control are not producing the expected results.

Mistake An error resulting from a faulty intention (contrast with lapse, slip).

Mode confusion (with respect to equipment operation) Mode confusion results from shortcomings in the user interface of a piece of equipment and is said to occur when:

- the operator of a piece of equipment believes the equipment is operating in a different one to the one in which it is really operating
- the operator does not know what mode the equipment is operating in.

Near miss An event or situation that could have resulted in an accident, injury, or illness, but did not, either by chance or through timely intervention. Near misses are 'free lessons' and should be prized as valuable learning opportunities.

Negligence Care that fell below the standard expected of physicians in their community.

Non-technical skills The cognitive and interpersonal skills needed to be a team member or a team leader in a safety-critical situation. The *cognitive skills* include those mental processes used for gaining and maintaining situation awareness, for solving problems, and making decisions. *Interpersonal skills* include communication and a range of behavioural activities associated with teamwork.

Operator A human factors term for any individual working in a 'high-risk industry' whose errors can lead to a fatal outcome (e.g. pilots, doctors, nurses, train drivers, chemical plant control room operatives, etc.).

Organizational error/accident An error that results from the way the work is organized rather than from lack of technical (medical) skills and knowledge. Thus a case of wrong side surgery is an organizational error (although the operation itself may be carried out with great surgical skill)

Patient safety The avoidance, prevention, and amelioration of adverse outcomes or injuries stemming from the processes of healthcare. These events include 'errors', 'deviations', and 'accidents'.

Perceptual narrowing A phenomenon where a subject's breadth of perception narrows in extremely stressful situations. As a result he may fail to notice stimuli suggesting that he has made the wrong mental model.

Preventability (of errors) Some types of error are easier to prevent than others. Organizations that initiate error management programmes invariably target the most preventable errors first before addressing the more difficult types of error.

Read back The repeating back of the essence of a message by its receiver in order that the sender can confirm that it has been correctly understood.

Red flag A situation that may constitute evidence of an incipient adverse situation.

Red rules Rules that must be followed to the letter. Any deviation from a red rule must bring work to a halt until compliance is achieved.

Risk consciousness A culture in which errors and systems failures are expected to occur at any time.

Risk management In the context of hospital operations, the term risk management usually refers to self-protective activities meant to prevent real or potential threats of financial loss due to accident, injury, or medical malpractice.

Root cause analysis A process for identifying the most basic or casual factor or factors that underlie variation in performance, including the occurrence of an adverse event.

Safety culture Safety culture and culture of safety are frequently encountered terms referring to a commitment to safety that permeates all levels of an organization, from front-line personnel to executive management. More specifically, 'safety culture' describes a number of features identified in studies of high reliability organizations outside of healthcare with exemplary performance with respect to safety. These features include:

- acknowledgment of the high-risk, error-prone nature of an organization's activities

- a blame-free environment where individuals are able to report errors or close calls without fear of reprimand or punishment

- an expectation of collaboration across ranks to seek solutions to vulnerabilities

- a willingness on the part of the organization to direct resources for addressing safety concerns.

Sentinel event (American term) A major accident. The choice of the word 'sentinel' reflects the egregiousness of the event and the likelihood that investigation of such events will reveal serious systems failures.

Situational awareness The relationship between an operator's mental model and the reality of the current operational situation. If that mental model is accurate in all essential elements, situational awareness is said to be high. If there is a significant difference between reality and the model, awareness is said to be lost.

Slip An unintended error of execution of a correctly intended action (contrast with lapse, mistake).

Standard operating procedures Precisely defined, systematic, and safe methods of carrying out tasks. Periodically revised in order to incorporate the lessons learned from accidents. They are designed to maximize an operator's situation awareness and to facilitate team resource management.

System A system is a collection of elements that function together to achieve some objective. The elements of the 'healthcare' system can be classified in one of four areas:

1 *Hardware*—tangible objects, such as equipment, medication, etc., but not including documentation.

2 *Liveware*—humans; clinicians, patients, support personnel, management.

3 *Software*—procedures, work schedules, policies, cultural values, documentation.

4 *Environment*—conditions that affect changes in the other elements, for example, long working hours that induce fatigue and reduced performance in clinicians.

Systems approach The concept that, although individuals make errors, the characteristics of the systems within which they work can make errors more likely and also more difficult to detect and correct. Further, the system approach takes the position that while individuals must be responsible for the quality of their work, more errors will be eliminated by focusing on systems than on individuals.

System failures Long-term situations that induce human error or inhibit error detection or prevention. These are usually associated with poor management.

Team resource management A process of interaction between the members of a team whereby each member of the team is empowered and encouraged to contribute in the most effective way to the task of the team. This can only take place if every member of the team fully understands their role within the group and how this role may vary depending the operational circumstances. Thus good team resource management requires agreed standard operating procedures.

Threat A long-standing situation or condition that is, in itself, either inherently dangerous or can induce the errors or loss of awareness. Most threats can be revealed by studying previous accident reports. Teams can work together to look for novel threats not previously associated with accidents but that are rendered more likely by new technologies or situations.

Threat management A systematic review of the risks that threaten to cause adverse incidents to patients or staff in a team, department, speciality, or other group. Best carried out as a preventative measure with wide involvement of professions and staff grades, to identify practical changes to systems and highlight area's where staff need particular caution or vigilance.

'Time outs' (American term) Planned periods of quiet and/or interdisciplinary discussion focused on ensuring that key procedural details have been addressed. For instance, protocols for ensuring correct site surgery often recommend a 'time out' to confirm the identification of the patient, the surgical procedure, site, and other key aspects, often stating them aloud for double-checking by other team members. In addition to avoiding major misidentification errors involving the patient or surgical site, such a time out ensures that all team members share the same 'game plan' so to speak. Taking the time to focus on listening and communicating the plans as a team can rectify miscommunications and misunderstandings before a procedure gets underway.

Usability testing This is a method by which representative users of a product are asked to perform certain tasks in an effort to measure the product's ease-of-use, task time, and the user's perception of the experience. Usability testing can be carried out using 'hi-tech' methods such as video cameras to observe operators or informally, with operators reporting their experiences with the equipment verbally or in writing usually in the form of a questionnaire.

User interface The user interface is those parts of a machine that the operator uses to interact with the machine. The user interface provides means of 'inputting', which allows the users to control the system, and 'output' by which the machine informs the users of the system status.

'Work-around' (American term)

Short-term changes to operational procedures made in order to continue work when problems such as missing documents or equipment encountered. Although 'work-arounds' are carried out for the best of motives they have been associated with serious adverse events.

Appendix 1: Initiating a safety-critical (verbal) communication (STAR)

S

Stop: Stop or a moment—remember that a misunderstood communication about a patient can be as harmful as a misdiagnosis or a medication error.

T

Think

—right time	Is this the right time to send this message?
—right person	Are you addressing the right person?
—right medium	What is the right medium for this message?
—relevant data	Do you have all relevant data to hand if the other party is likely to ask questions?
—opening phrase	Do you need to use an opening phrase that makes the purpose of the message absolutely clear?
—structure	Consider if it would it be helpful to compose the message using one of the following structures:

- NEED/DATA/ACTION (for general messages)
- I-S B A R (for messages about a patient's condition)

Think how your message could possibly be misunderstood—be risk conscious

A

Articulate clearly: Take a breath so that you are able to voice the entire message clearly.

If possible, make eye contact with the other party.

Using the other party's name is usually helpful.

Use straightforward words. Consider avoiding the use of abbreviations, esoteric terminology

R

Response/read back: Observe how the message is received, particularly the body language of the receiver.

Listen to the read back.

If there is any doubt that the message has been successfully passed, re-send the message using different words or message structure.

Appendix 2: I-SBAR—to describe a (deteriorating) patient's condition

I

Identify yourself, unit, patient, ward and/or room number.

S

Situation: 'The problem is persistent, heavy haematuria …'

- ◆ Briefly state the problem, what is it, when it happened or started, and how severe.

B

Background: 'There is a background history of bladder cancer… '—
Pertinent background information related to the situation.
   You could include the following:

- ◆ The working diagnosis and date of admission: 'The patient was admitted yesterday having had recent confirmation of a recurrent bladder tumour at cystoscopy … '
- ◆ List of current medications, allergies, IV fluids, and blood results
- ◆ Most recent vital signs: 'I think the patient is haemodynamically unstable despite having had iv fluids and 3 units of blood. The pulse rate is … and the blood pressure is … '
- ◆ Blood results: provide the date and time test was done and results of previous tests for comparison
- ◆ Other clinical information.

A

Assessment: 'My assessment is that the patient has uncontrolled bleeding … '

R

Recommendation: 'I think the patient needs to come to theatres within the next hour … '

- ◆ 'I need you to come to see the patient now'

Remember: Document the change in the patient's condition and this communication.

Appendix 3: General patient safety tools

- *'Read back'*. Repeat back verbal safety critical messages so that correct understanding can be assured. Replace any pronouns with the actual name of the patient or medication, etc.
- *'Summarize plans'*. Sum up discussions about a patient's treatment plan to ensure there are no misunderstandings. Ensure everyone knows who is doing what.
- 'Active identification'
  - ask patients to give you their name and date of birth.
  - ensure that the parties to a communication are identified to each other (particularly over the telephone or where the parties have not met before).
- *Stop* and *think* before initiating a verbal communication (see Appendix 1).
  - when constructing a *safety-critical message* it may be helpful to *structure* your message.
  - when describing a critical patient condition consider using the *I-SBAR* protocol—*identification, situation, background, assessment, recommendation.* (see Appendix 2)
- *'Speak up'*. If something seems to be going wrong but the situation is not being recognized or acknowledged by other team members, *speak up*.
  - use an alert phrase to draw the attention of the team to 'red flags' (the symptoms and signs of an impending error) (see Appendix 4)
  - in extremis, use the *PACE* approach

Before carrying out an unfamiliar procedure *stop* for a moment and *think* about the potential negative outcomes. You should *act* cautiously and *review* the result, looking for the evidence that the action has been successful or unsuccessful.

Be honest

- If you have made a mistake.
- If you do not understand a message or an instruction, ask for clarification.
- If you do not know what is going on, draw uncertainties to the attention of the team.

Participate in critical incident reporting programmes

- Report your errors, describing how you were induced to make the error.
- Report error-inducing situations.
- Report unserviceable equipment and poor equipment design.
- Report poorly designed procedures, missing documents, and so on.

Be aware of

- The theory of the *aetiology of adverse events.*
- Activities that have been associated with *irreversible errors* in the past.
- Error-inducing situations such as *'changes of plan'.*
- The possibility of *'mind-lock', confirmation bias,* and *unconscious inferences.*
- The possibility of a undetected and malevolent *coincidence.*
- The importance of the precise *taxonomy* of error and human factors.

Safety-critical communications

Message structure

To ensure maximum effectiveness, a communication whose content might not be expected or might be misunderstood by its recipient should have two or three of the following elements:

1	2	3
Need (purpose)	Data	Action
—state the 'need' that the message is intended to address	—give the essential piece of data relating to the subject matter	—clearly state what action you think should be carried out and by whom
—or use an 'opening' phrase		
—or an 'alert' phrase		

Opening phrases	Alert phrases
'So, to sum up then the plan now is … '	'I need a little clarity … '
'This is an emergency … '	'I need to understand why … '
'This is urgent … '	'I haven't a clue what's going on … '
'This is a change of plan … '	'I think we have some red flags here … '
'This is non-standard … '	'I am not happy about this … '
'This is not what you are expecting, but … '	
'This is a correction … '	
'I could not help noticing that … '	'Something's wrong … '
'I need to confirm that … '	'I need you to come to see the patient now'
'I need to understand why … '	'You must listen … '
'I need reassurance … '	'STOP NOW'

If you receive a safety-critical message it might be useful to 'decode' it by attempting to assess what '*need*' it was intended to address. If this is not clear, ask for clarification. Is the *data* in the message valid? Is it clear who is to carry out any *actions* suggested in the message?

Useful things to say

To create a *candid atmosphere* in the team

- 'If, at any point, you think I am making a mistake, you may be right. Please tell me straight away'
- 'If you spot something you think I have missed, please tell me straight away'

To request *input in a crisis* where situation awareness may have been lost

- 'Can anyone think of anything that we are not doing that we need to do?'
- 'I haven't got a clue what's going on here. Any ideas anyone?'

Note:
It might be useful to learn these sentences off by heart in advance because the stress of the crisis may reduce the available cognitive resources to construct these requests at the time.

Appendix 4: Red flags (the symptoms and signs of an impending error)

If you are about to carry out a procedure or you are carrying out a procedure where any of the following situations may occur or are occurring, you should draw this to the attention of the rest of the team.

1 Ambiguities/anomalies/conflicting information or expectations/surprises.

2 Broken communications/inconclusive discussions.

3 Confusion/loss of awareness/uncertainties.

4 Missing information/missing steps/missing equipment/incomplete briefings.

5 Departures from normal procedures or practices/'work arounds'/ 'helping out'.

6 Fixation/tunnel vision/preoccupation.

7 Changes of plan.

8 Time distortion/event runaway.

9 Unease/fear.

10 Denial/stress/inaction.

11 Juniors cut short.

12 Alarm bells.

If departures from normal practices, changes of plan or missing information are inevitable in your current operational situation, be aware of the greater risk of error. Brief team members to look for other red flags.

Verbalization

On identifying one or more unresolved red flags you should make a remark to the effect of: 'I think we have some red flags here'.

Speaking up strategy: PACE (Probe, Alert, Challenge, Emergency)

Level 1: Probe

Ask a question to find out why the other team member(s) seem to have a different mental model. If there is a suggestion of a 'red flag' situation you have the right to ask for clarification.

- 'I need to understand why ...'

Level 2: Alert

If the question is not answered appropriately and your concerns are still unresolved, you should alert the team or team leader to the potential danger that you think the present course of action might bring.

- 'I am not happy...'

Level 3: Challenge

If the team leader continues on the course of action, you should adopt a very assertive tone and state that in his view the present situation is unsafe and challenge the team leader to change the plan:

- 'You must listen ...'

Level 4: Emergency

It is the duty of any team member to take control of a situation or halt a procedure when the previous levels of the PACE strategy have not been responded to adequately or where a definite danger is identified.

- 'STOP NOW'

Note: The use of the other team member's name when addressing them is usually highly effective—but do not turn this into a personal battle.

Criticize the action, not the individual.

Index